Brief interventions with bereaved children

Oxford University Press makes no representation, express or implied, that the drug dosages in this book are correct. Readers must therefore always check the product information and clinical procedures with the most up to date published product information and data sheets provided by the manufacturers and the most recent codes of conduct and safety regulations. The authors and the publishers do not accept responsibility or legal liability for any errors in the text or for the misuse or misapplication of material in this work.

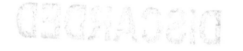

Brief interventions with bereaved children

Edited by

Barbara Monroe
Chief Executive
St Christopher's Hospice
London, UK

and

Frances Kraus
Candle Project Leader
St Christopher's Hospice
London, UK

OXFORD
UNIVERSITY PRESS

OXFORD
UNIVERSITY PRESS

Great Clarendon Street, Oxford OX2 6DP

Oxford University Press is a department of the University of Oxford.
It furthers the University's objective of excellence in research, scholarship,
and education by publishing worldwide in

Oxford New York

Auckland Cape Town Dar es Salaam Hong Kong Karachi
Kuala Lumpur Madrid Melbourne Mexico City Nairobi
New Delhi Shanghai Taipei Toronto

With offices in

Argentina Austria Brazil Chile Czech Republic France Greece
Guatemala Hungary Italy Japan South Korea Poland Portugal
Singapore Switzerland Thailand Turkey Ukraine Vietnam

Oxford is a registered trade mark of Oxford University Prss
in the UK and in certain other countries

Published in the United States
by Oxford University Press Inc., New York

A catalogue record for this title is available from the British Library

ISBN 0 19 852909 0 (Pbk)

10 9 8 7 6 5 4 3 2

Typeset by Cepha Imaging Private Ltd., Bangalore, India
Printed in Great Britain
on acid-free paper by
Biddles Ltd., King's Lynn, Norfolk

Foreword

What makes this book so valuable is that Barbara Monroe and her colleagues have brought together the very latest in individual, group, and community approaches, thoroughly informed by the cutting edge of practice and research in this gradually emerging area of children's bereavement. Its unique contribution is the authors' solid grounding in actual practice with children in many different service sites, each chapter providing several case examples that give voice to the grief of children and adolescents as well as adults. The work of the Childhood Bereavement Network described indicates the importance of a national educational and advocacy agenda with the goal of increasing the accessibility, quality, comprehensiveness, and continuity of these services.

A number of critical challenges in providing services for bereaved children are addressed through the descriptions of intervention models the authors have found effective. Such challenges include: 1) timing issues in relation to type of death and length of the recovery process; 2) the interaction between psychological, social, and ecological factors in bereaved children; and 3) the use of multiple, often simultaneous interventions.

Time

The trajectory of the dying process and the trajectory of the recovery process should influence the type and timing of interventions proposed for children. In the research we conducted on children who confront an expected death of a parent to cancer, we found they experienced their highest levels of anxiety and depression before the parent's death, with a fairly rapid decrease in these stress levels after the death occurred (Christ 2000). This finding strongly suggests that the period before the death is an opportune time for intervention, offering possibilities of lowering distress by clarifying information and communication, encouraging final conversations, reducing family conflict, and arranging for continuing follow up. Our findings concur with the author of the chapter on pre-bereavement work that preparatory work, however difficult, is valued by parents and especially children who so often said 'I was surprised when Dad died, but I was prepared, Mom told me it would happen'. Conversely, when children were not given preparatory information that was known to adults, their loss of trust in the parent and anger at being unprepared when the loss was clearly inevitable complicated their bereavement.

Sudden death is also addressed in innovative and helpful ways in several chapters. These include suicide, homicide, and accidents, as well as the increasing natural and man-made disasters associated with regional and worldwide conflicts. The book acknowledges the need to address both trauma and grief responses during bereavement. Interventions must take account of the impact of the loss of the person, but also the fear, sometimes terror, surrounding the particular circumstances of the death and its aftermath. Those who have experienced the sudden death of a loved one often comprise an underserved population. Many such families may have no previous connection with health professionals.

The timing or the trajectory of recovery also affects the type of help that is offered. Brief treatments are suggested in this book within the context of a 'warranty' or guarantee of professional availability for later problems that may emerge. Some authors describe multiple services reaching out to offer many ways of 'staying connected' with programs even when individual sessions are not needed or wanted. This approach is supported by findings from our own and others' bereavement research. Brief packages of interventions are more valued by families if they provide some form of continuing care or connection for families. Children express their grief more briefly than adults, but their responses seem to continue over a longer period of time. They may react to later reminders of the loss, changes in their own cognitive and emotional capacity may bring up new concerns, and new developmental tasks that are complicated by the absence of a parent or sibling may become powerful reminders of the loss.

Interaction between psychological, social, and ecological factors

Rather than focusing on one conceptual model and approach to intervention, the book presents multiple approaches implemented within an ecological systems perspective. This is especially important for children as the developmental, social, and interpersonal dimensions of their bereavement are powerfully interactive with their internal experience. The authors also firmly adopt a family and community focus. This focus acknowledges research that has established a strong relationship between the primary caregiver's competence with children during bereavement and children's ability to cope with such stress. Innovative group and volunteer programmes for caregivers are also described. Coping with bereavement not only requires that children manage intense emotions, but also that the family must reconstitute a 'new normal' for itself, redefining roles and relationships without the day-to-day presence of the person who died. Children also need to develop a satisfying life experience within this new family and community context.

The critical importance of the school having teachers who are knowledgeable about providing education and support to bereaved children, as well as receiving help with their own reactions to such tragedies, matches our own experience in work with families of firefighters killed in the 9/11 attacks on the World Trade Center. Teachers and school guidance counsellors can help to normalize a student's experience through group and individual contacts. However, they need education and training to be effective and to prevent their own emotional overload. We learned through this very public tragedy how the impact of ongoing local and national events created stressful reminders for bereaved children over several years.

Use of multiple, often simultaneous, interventions at different locations

Most impressive in this book is the broad range of interventions and special techniques described for work with bereaved children. The use of the Internet, telephone, and newer technologies, children's activity groups, volunteer programmes, and self-help groups for caregivers are all vital components of an effective programme. The chapter on techniques shows inventiveness in response to the many challenges of working with bereaved children. The authors describe the use of play, arts and crafts, understanding externalizing behaviours, accepting children's need to have fun, appreciating their need to distance themselves from the grief at times, to enjoy positive feelings and pleasurable experiences even in the midst of tragedy, and to understand the normalcy of their grief reactions and their transient nature.

Only in the past two decades has childhood bereavement been studied systematically and reported direct responses from children. In part, this is due to the very moving nature of this work as one listens to children's poignant yearning for the lost family member. The editors of this volume, who are acknowledged international leaders in this field, present their work with sensitivity and compassion for the stresses families are confronting. It is a remarkable accomplishment and a must read for all engaged in this important work. Having worked in this field for many years, I too have learned much from this book.

Grace Christ, DSW
Associate Professor
Columbia University School of Social Work
Director, Fire Department of NYC Family Guidance Programme

Reference

Christ G (2000). *Healing children's grief: surviving a parent's death from cancer.* Oxford: Oxford University Press.

Preface

At a conference I attended recently on childhood bereavement a participant questioned whether, given the contradictory nature of much of the available research data, there was really anything valid we could say about what helps children and their families and carers. This book has been written out of a profound conviction that whilst many questions remain unanswered, there is much that we do know. Children and young people need to have their experiences acknowledged and support to find ways of articulating their story and to regain some sense of control and confidence in a world that they often experience as chaotic. They need opportunities to remember and where possible a chance to meet others with similar experiences. Support from close friends appears significant. Help needs to be delivered in the context of children's families, existing social relationships, and communities, so that these networks are enabled to support over time children whose responses to their loss will change and develop over time.

There is incomplete but developing evidence that the interplay between reactions to grief and other risk factors can lead to negative outcomes for bereaved children, particularly among children who are already vulnerable, both during childhood and later in adult life. The experience of bereavement also seems to have the potential to give some children an increased sense of resourcefulness, maturity, and self-esteem. Research clearly indicates that children's adaptation to bereavement depends much on how their parent or carer manages to support them.

There are inevitable limits to direct service provision and need will always outstrip available specialist resource. The provision of less intensive interventions can make sense as part of a preventive, public health approach. Flexible and accessible short-term services delivered at the right time can underpin the strength of bereaved children, young people, and their families, supporting their recovery rather than pathologising the grief process. Innovative methods of contact will help to extend service reach and respond to individual choice. There is no one-size service that fits all. Every writer in this volume believes that all children and their families and carers have the right to appropriate, culturally sensitive basic information, advice, and support. A few will need much more.

This book resonates with the concept of resilience and the importance of working with the strength and possibilities of children, young people, and their families, rather than merely identifying their problems. It is vital that capacity and resource is developed amongst the communities and professional networks in which children already live and in which they can grow and develop, even in the presence of tragic loss. It is also important that bereavement in children and young people is integrated into all aspects of government policy and national service planning.

Society remains afraid of death and adults' fear and silence can leave children's grief invisible and unsupported. We have a responsibility to ensure that bereaved children are neither forgotten, nor their needs left unmet. This underlines the importance of helping parents and families to help their children. Death and loss are part of life. However much we desire to protect children we cannot create for them a world in which these experiences do not exist. Together we can offer children support so that in confronting and learning about death, loss, and grief, they develop the emotional capacity and intelligence that will sustain them for the rest of their lives.

B.M.

Contents

List of contributors

Isobel Bremner, Candle Project Worker, St Christopher's Hospice, London, UK.

Gillian Chowns, Senior Specialist Palliative Care Social Worker, East Berks Macmillan Palliative Care Team, King Edward VII Hospital, Windsor, UK and Senior Lecturer in Palliative Care, Oxford Brookes University, Oxford, UK.

Ann Dent, Honorary Research Fellow and Chair, Bereavement Research Forum, Department of Child Health, Bristol University, Bristol, UK.

Atle Dyregrov, Director and Clinical Psychologist, Centre for Crisis Psychology, Bergen, Norway.

Kari Dyregrov, Researcher and Sociologist, Centre for Crisis Psychology, Bergen, Norway.

Julie Ellison, Detective Sergeant, Metropolitan Police, Diversity Directorate, New Scotland Yard, London, UK.

Peta Hemmings, Senior Practitioner, Barnardo's, Newcastle upon Tyne, UK.

Frances Kraus, Candle Project Leader, St Christopher's Hospice, London, UK

Christine Pentland, Director, SeeSaw, Oxford, UK.

Louise Rowling, Associate Professor, Faculty of Education and Social Work, University of Sydney, Sydney, Australia.

Stewart Sinclair, Co-founder and Co-leader of Candle Parent Carer Support Group, St Christopher's Hospice, London, UK.

Peter Speck, Visiting Fellow and Former NHS Health Care Chaplain, Faculty of Medicine, University of Southampton, Southampton, UK.

Julie Stokes, Chief Executive and Consultant Clinical Psychologist, Winston's Wish, Cheltenham, UK.

Di Stubbs, Helpline and Web Co-ordinator, Winston's Wish, Cheltenham, UK.

Patsy Way, Candle Project Worker, St Christopher's Hospice, London, UK.

Sarah Willis, Director, Childhood Bereavement Network, Nottingham, UK.

William Yule, Professor of Applied Child Psychology, Institute of Psychology, The Maudsley Hospital, London, UK.

Chapter 1

Work with bereaved children

Sarah Willis

Every day in the United Kingdom, around 50 children are bereaved of a parent (Stokes 2004).

This is a sad and shocking statistic because it reveals the existence of a largely unacknowledged group of vulnerable children and young people who are coping every day with a profound experience of personal loss. Moreover this statistic does not include children who are bereaved of a sister or brother, a grandparent or other close relative, or a neighbour, friend, or teacher. If it did these figures would be far higher.

Over the last 20 years in the United Kingdom, the needs of bereaved children, young people and their families have been increasingly recognized, evident in the steady growth in the support and services available to bereaved children and young people. This growth has been stimulated by a number of factors. The experience of working with families where a death was expected led many hospices to develop skills and resources to meet the needs of children facing bereavement. In more recent years they have increasingly used these services as a springboard to develop special children's programmes that also respond to the needs of children bereaved through sudden death. In Rolls and Payne's study (2003) of current service provision, adult and children's hospices made up 44% ($n = 40$) of the survey cohort. Winston's Wish, an early example of a community-based grief support programme for children in Gloucestershire, was established in 1992 and has been used as a model for many other similar service developments. Research also played its part in stimulating service development, particularly the work of Dora Black from the 1980s onwards and Silverman and Worden's Harvard Child Bereavement study and its dissemination through Worden's widely sold book 'Children and Grief: When a Parent Dies' (1996).

Service developments stimulated the production of materials, videos, books, and literature for professionals, families, and children. An early example was 'Someone Special Has Died', a booklet written specifically for children and published by St Christopher's Hospice in 1989. It was quickly translated into 8 languages, selling over 50,000 English copies in its first six years of publication. Ann Couldrick had written a booklet for adults, 'Grief and Bereavement: Understanding Children' in 1988. Marge Heegaard's workbook for children 'When Someone Very Special Dies' (1988) inspired others to produce similar books. Books for practitioners followed, including Dyregrov's 'Grief in Children: A Handbook for Adults' published in 1991 and 'Interventions with Bereaved Children' edited by Smith and Pennells and published in 1995.

Increased awareness led to a demand for more training for professionals and volunteers working with or coming into contact with bereaved children, including health and social care professionals, members of the clergy, teachers, Police Family Liaison officers, and youth workers. For example, at the time of writing, the Candle Children's Project at St Christopher's had trained 900 Metropolitan Police Family Liaison Officers. Considerable basic training opportunities are now available to anyone working with children and young people. Again hospices often took the lead in the early development of short courses and key in capturing professional engagement was the 1991 video 'That Morning I Went to School' produced by the Northampton Child and Family Consultation Service which briefly and graphically demonstrated the needs of children and the extent to which the adult world had overlooked them. A significant advance was the launch in the United Kingdom of a new University-validated course for practitioners already experienced in the field. The innovative Undergraduate Diploma and Postgraduate Certificate in Child Bereavement is to commence in September 2004 and has been developed in partnership by St Christopher's Hospice and Help the Hospices in consultation with a range of interested agencies and individuals.

Bereavement support services for children have evolved in a variety of ways, in response to needs identified by the individuals and agencies working with bereaved families but also to demand from families themselves. For example:

- as extensions to existing adult bereavement support or counselling services;
- as extensions to existing hospice-based adult bereavement support services;
- as innovative, new models of service provision, e.g., residential camps;
- as new service initiatives stimulated by local demand, both professional and service user led.

The present situation

A recent study to identify the location, range, and type of childhood bereavement service provision in the United Kingdom [Rolls and Payne 2003], describes service provision as 'a diverse and complex tapestry … in terms of location, type of services, service organization, funding arrangements, and interventions offered.' Different children's bereavement services across the United Kingdom have different referral criteria and some only provide support to specific groups. A broad distinction can be made between 'restricted' and 'open access' services.

Restricted access services usually offer bereavement support services to select groups of children, who are usually already known to the host organization or service (often a hospice or palliative care team). For example, a child whose relative has died from cancer or other terminal illness whilst under the care of the local hospice or palliative care team would usually be able to access support pre/post bereavement from the specialist family and bereavement support service within the hospice. However, this support and/or support services might not be available to a child living within the same locality but with no connection to the hospice or palliative care team, whose parent, sibling, other relative or friend had died unexpectedly, for instance, in a road traffic collision or by suicide.

In contrast, an open access service generally offers a range of support and services to bereaved children and young people whatever the type/circumstances of the death (unexpected or anticipated) and whatever their relationship to the dead person. The only barriers to access are usually those of geographical boundaries or restrictions set on the age range catered for by the service.

Across the United Kingdom there is currently no consistency or standardization in service provision and access to services varies enormously. A recent mapping exercise (Childhood Bereavement Network 2003*a*) identified a number of counties in England where no open access service could be found.

A key division in the experience of bereaved children and families occurs between those bereavements which have been anticipated (e.g. a death from cancer) and those that are unexpected (e.g. a death in a road traffic collision). When a death is anticipated through a terminal illness, information, guidance, and support is usually easier to access. Following the death, further guidance and support is usually made available to family members by the same institution or team, primarily to enable the adults to support the bereaved children. Staff within the palliative care team or hospice social work/bereavement departments often take on a mediating or advocacy role on behalf of bereaved families. This may involve, for example, supporting the family and child/ren through the process of informing their schools of the death; providing advice to teachers and ancillary staff; sharing resources.

Children's hospices offer a comprehensive range of pre/post bereavement support services to siblings and parents. Irregular contact may be maintained for many years, for as long as the support is required.

When a death is unexpected it is often extremely difficult for children and families to get the support they need, in both the short and the long term. Immediately following the death, in addition to the family and friends, support may be offered by various professionals: a member of the clergy, the family doctor, funeral director, health visitor, or school staff. If the death was violent and traumatic – a murder, road traffic collision, or suicide – support may also be offered by the police, Victim Support, social workers or a self-help group such as Support after Murder and Manslaughter (SAMM). In some cases, the traumatic nature and circumstances of the death or deaths may lead to a short-term input from educational psychologists. Later, the child or children may also be offered a referral to the local Child and Adolescent Mental Health Service, although some waiting lists are long.

However, in the absence of a designated professional or local agency with a remit to provide ongoing bereavement care within a community, children and families who are bereaved without warning can find themselves unable to identify the advice and support they need, particularly in the longer term. Children and young people revisit the impact of their bereavement at different stages as they grow into adulthood. They sometimes find that teachers and other professionals have unrealistic expectations about the speed of grief resolution. One young man explained; 'I still get upset sometimes ... break down and cry. It's not just like it was before ... you have to explain to them – it's not okay; you're still upset. It doesn't just go away after a month or a couple of weeks or so ...' (Childhood Bereavement Network 2002).

Both open and restricted access services will usually offer support at four different levels to bereaved children, their families and other caregivers, including professional carers such as teachers, health visitors, and school nurses:

- Information: literature, website, e-mail, signposting
- Guidance: telephone advice and support from trained staff; family assessments; training and/or supervision sessions for professionals and volunteers
- Support: direct one-to-one support work with bereaved children, their families and other caregivers and/or group activities and social events
- At a fourth level, if suitably qualified staff are employed within the service, in-depth counselling or a therapeutic intervention may be offered to the bereaved child, or a referral may be made to a local Child and Adolescent Mental Health Service team or other specialized service.

The range of services and resources that are now available to bereaved children and families through the various specialized services include:

- A series of one-to-one sessions for the bereaved child or young person with a member of staff, either paid or unpaid;
- befriending or buddy schemes, where trained volunteers offer support individually tailored to the needs of the child or young person to whom they are linked;
- social events;
- access to networks of similarly bereaved families who can provide mutual emotional, practical, and social support;
- occasional and regular group meetings for adults and children where experiences and feelings can be shared and strategies for coping developed;
- weekend events or residential camps where time is set aside to talk, grieve, and celebrate the life of the person who has died as well as taking part in fun activities;
- memorial events, often held around Christmas;
- interactive websites, sometimes including message boards;
- newsletters in which children and young people can share their experiences and feelings;
- e-mail support;
- telephone helplines;
- a variety of printed resources, including postcards, leaflets, and posters.

A model of care is being developed for bereaved children, their families and other caregivers which:

- is community based;
- aims to provide preventative rather than reactive support to bereaved children and families;
- is non-stigmatizing and acknowledges the bereaved child as grieving and not ill;
- seeks to enable bereaved children and young people to cope with death as a normal life event and manage grief as a normal reaction to loss;

- primarily aims to offer holistic, supportive care and attention;
- offers a range of services which aim to facilitate and respond to the individual needs of bereaved children within the context of their families, schools, and as part of their wider life in the community (Stokes *et al.* 1999).

The Childhood Bereavement Network

In 1998, under the umbrella of the National Association of Bereavement Services, a multi-agency collaborative project was set up, 'to improve the quality and range of bereavement support for children, young people, and their families in the United Kingdom.' The launch of the Childhood Bereavement Project (CBP) reflected awareness within the field of bereavement care that a co-ordinated approach was needed to ensure that all children affected by the death of someone significant in their lives could easily access high quality information, guidance, and support.

In 1998, the CBP began a collaboration with Marie Curie Cancer Care on the organization of a national conference on bereavement in childhood, which was ultimately held in March, 2000. To inform the design of the conference programme, a series of regional consultation meetings were arranged to enable consultation with practitioners working with bereaved children and families. By early 1999, the Childhood Bereavement Project had been awarded a three year grant by The Diana, Princess of Wales Memorial Fund to create a national 'network' to link together support services for bereaved children and establish standards and codes of good practice. Therefore, the series of consultation meetings also aimed to collect information to feed into the new CBP project and gain a broad perspective on what were perceived to be key principles for best practice in bereavement care for children. Subsequently, from 1999 to 2002, CBP Area Groups were established and meetings were held twice yearly in 12 locations around the United Kingdom. These meetings also provided an opportunity to deliver training events.

The first sessions of CBP Area Group meetings offered extensive opportunities for face-to-face consultation and discussion between practitioners on the proposed 'Guidelines for Best Practice' and a proposed structure for the new national network. Further consultation and feedback was achieved by the circulation of a Consultation Document, with around 800 copies of the document being sent to interested individuals and organizations throughout the UK.

The 'Childhood Bereavement Network' was launched as a subscription scheme at the first CBN conference in Birmingham in June, 2001 together with a CBN 'Belief Statement' and the 'Guidelines for Best Practice'. The publication of the CBN 'Guidelines for Best Practice' represented a significant achievement in terms of achieving consensus in the field. The challenge for the project was to introduce an inclusive but robust framework which would promote and encourage good practice rather than impose unrealistic mandatory standards. It was recognized that the 'Guidelines' could only represent the first stage in what will inevitably be a lengthy process of defining and validating the range of work which had developed in an ad hoc, although innovative manner, within the voluntary sector.

As a 'virtual' network of service providers and practitioners, hosted by the National Children's Bureau, the CBN continues to grow and expand its role as a membership

GUIDELINES FOR BEST PRACTICE

Safety

- Is there a documented policy to ensure the overall safety of children using your service/s? Does this policy encompass the whole range of work undertaken by paid/voluntary staff e.g. individual/group work, transport by volunteers, home visits?
- Does the policy incorporate a set procedure for the recruitment of paid staff and volunteers?
- Do paid and voluntary staff receive training and supervision to ensure the overall safety of children using your service?
- Do you work within the legislative framework and guidance, specifically the Children Act 1989, *Working Together to Safeguard Children* documents; *Safe from Harm* (Home Office), *Duty to Care* (DHSS Northern Ireland) and the Children (Scotland) Act 1995?
- Is there a documented policy on confidentiality? Is this reviewed on a regular basis and agreed with paid/voluntary staff?
- Is there a documented policy to ensure the personal safety of paid/voluntary staff? Is this policy reviewed and evaluated regularly in consultation with all staff?

Practice Context

- Are the principles embodied in the CBN Belief Statement incorporated into your practice and the service/s you provide? Do you regularly review your approach to your work? As an organisation, do you consult with paid/voluntary staff during this process?
- Is your documented policy on confidentiality fully discussed and agreed with the individual child, the parent/s, other family members and caregivers?
- Is there a documented health and safety policy?
- Are there procedures in place to ensure data protection?
- Are documented policies and procedures reviewed regularly to comply with legal requirements?
- Is your service appropriately resourced? Do you have reliable access to a safe space, room or premises? Do you have a budget to buy equipment?

Quality and Accountability

- Do you have procedures to enable you to monitor, evaluate and review the service/s you provide on a regular basis?
- Do you regularly undertake a needs assessment to review the appropriateness of your work or service/s? Do you liaise with users, key referral agencies, staff and other professionals working in your catchment area regarding any proposed service development? Do you have a procedure to ensure effective liaison with other local, regional or national organisations offering similar services?
- Is there a documented policy to ensure that all paid/voluntary staff are appropriately trained to work with bereaved children, their families and other caregivers? Are training needs regularly reviewed? Are all paid/voluntary staff offered regular opportunities to update their skills? Do you have a training budget?
- Is there a documented policy on supervision? Are all paid/voluntary staff appropriately supervised? Are paid/voluntary staff consulted on a regular basis to agree their supervision needs?
- Do you encourage feedback on your service from users, key referral agencies and professionals? Is there a documented and accessible complaints procedure for users, key referral agencies, paid/voluntary staff and the public?
- Do you have a statement of purpose or mission statement plus clear aims to define the remit of your service? Is there a business plan, including a funding strategy to ensure the sustainability of your service? Do you publish and circulate an annual report to key referral agencies and users?
- Is there a written definition of your service/s, which clearly sets out details of the information, guidance and support you offer? Is this regularly reviewed and updated? Within the remit of your service, is this information circulated to key referral agencies and potential users in the form of a publicity leaflet?

Equality

- Is there a documented and proactive equal opportunities policy?
- Do you regularly undertake a needs assessment to review the accessibility and appropriateness of your service/s in terms of equality of opportunity?
- Do you regularly review your service/s to identify and amend any anti-discriminatory practice?
- Are you able to respond to the needs of bereaved minority ethinic children, especially in terms of language?
- Are you able to respond to the needs of bereaved disabled children or those with learning disabilities?
- Do you liaise with other organisations to raise awareness of the needs of bereaved children, their families and other caregivers?

Childhood Bereavement Network, 8 Wakley Street, London EC1V 7QE Tel: 020 7843 6309 Fax: 020 7837 1439 e-mail: cbn@ncb.org.uk

Fig. 1.1 Childhood Bereavement Network Guidelines.

and co-ordinating body. To date, more than 260 organizations and individuals have subscribed to the Childhood Bereavement Network and endorsed the CBN 'Belief Statement' and 'Guidelines for Best Practice' as a criterion of their membership.

In 2002, the Childhood Bereavement Network was commissioned by the Children and Young People's Unit at the United Kingdom Government Department of Education and Skills to undertake a mapping exercise to identify open access children's bereavement support services in England and compile an online Directory.

More than 800 questionnaires were sent out by the CBN to contacts throughout England; for example to children's bereavement services, hospices, church groups, funeral directors, and palliative care teams, asking respondents to self-assess their status as either an open access or restricted service and complete the questionnaire accordingly. Contacts were also asked to supply information about any other open access services in their locality and to pass on copies of the questionnaire. For the purposes of the survey, an open access service was defined as a service that would offer support to any bereaved child or young person:

♦ whatever the type/circumstances of the death (unexpected or anticipated);

♦ whatever their relationship to the dead person;

♦ whatever their culture, beliefs, and religion;

♦ and with the only barriers to access being geographical boundaries.

The survey identified 47 open access specialized bereavement support services for children in England. (This did not include those local branches of Cruse Bereavement Care which offer support to children and young people.)

In common with the Clara Burgess Charity Research Project survey (Rolls and Payne 2003), the CBN mapping exercise confirmed that there is no standard organizational structure or model for service provision to bereaved children and young people. This has important implications for future strategy on service development. Services appear to have developed as a reflection of specific local or regional needs, including the location, cultural mix, and the skills base of those involved in setting up the service. However, it appears significant that 40 of the services were registered charities or operated under the umbrella of a larger organization (often a hospice) which was a registered charity. There was no consistent criterion, in terms of age, for access to the different types of service nor consistency in terms of catchment areas for services. The mapping exercise led to the compilation of the CBN Directory of Open Access Support Services for Bereaved Children and Young People and its launch as an online resource for families and professionals seeking information, guidance, and support. The Directory, which is constantly updated to reflect changes in service provision and the development of new services, may be accessed on www.ncb.org.uk/cbn/directory. The Directory aims to increase awareness of the range of accessible, specialized bereavement support services for children and young people in England and to enable easy access to a choice of information, guidance, and support. In due course, the scope of the Directory will be extended into Northern Ireland, Scotland, and Wales.

The services in the Directory can be contacted directly for information, guidance, and support by anyone who is caring for or working with a bereaved child or young person or, in many instances, by the bereaved child or young person themselves. The Directory only contains details of open access services for bereaved children and young people although it is recognized that there are many other types of specialized children's bereavement support services in England that are currently restricted in terms of accessibility. In due course, the Directory will be extended in scope to include these different categories of service. All the services included in the Directory have subscribed to the CBN. In instances where there is no local service listed, details of national telephone helplines and services are included.

Another consequence of the CBN mapping exercise was that gaps in service provision for bereaved children and young people in England were identified. In 2003, to promote service growth, the CBN applied for and received further funding in the form of a three-year strategic grant from the Community Fund for development work in England. A key objective of the project work is to provide a consultancy service and to utilize the resource of the CBN membership to encourage and mentor open access service development for bereaved children in the areas of need identified during the mapping exercise. An information pack and online resource will be created to support the development of new services.

Mainstream funding for children's bereavement support services is still only provided in pockets around the United Kingdom and achieving sustainable streams of funding for services remains a challenge. The majority of the services are voluntary organizations and the survey reported by Rolls and Payne (2003) shows sources of funding to be diverse; donations and legacies, fund-raising, grants, income generation through activities such as training, and sponsorship.

Another strand of work to be achieved by the CBN under the terms of its new grant is the expansion into explicit detail of its existing 'Guidelines for Best Practice'. Funding is also being sought to develop a bespoke self-assessment quality assurance scheme for children's bereavement support services.

The future

Over the past 20 years, the sphere of bereavement care for children has changed immensely. There is a much greater awareness of the needs of children and young people affected by the death of someone close to them and policies, services, and skills are gradually being developed to respond to these needs. The work of specialist bereavement support services is now widely recognized and valued. New and different types of service are being developed at local and national level, for example interactive websites, school grief support programmes, and telephone helplines.

Bereaved children and young people are increasingly consulted and participate in the development of new services, and are encouraged to voice their opinions and speak about their experiences. They are involved in the production of resources of all kinds. The CBN has produced a series of videos involving children and young people as part of its Video Talkshop project, funded by Children in Need, and in 2004, after consultation, will publish *Guidelines for Participation* to encourage good and innovative practice in this area.

However, despite these positive advances, challenges remain for those working in child bereavement care, seeking to develop support networks and services for bereaved children. In the United Kingdom, despite a generally benevolent view that bereavement support and services are on the whole beneficial, they are not a priority in terms of national and local policy making and the allocation of funding and resources. There is no significant recognition by policy makers and professional communities that bereaved children are vulnerable and might potentially, in negative circumstances and without adequate support, become 'at risk'. For example a recent ChildLine report (Cross 2002), highlighted some of the more extreme experiences of bereaved children and young people:

- 'We are worried about Dad – he doesn't wash, he's always in the pub. I try to wash and iron like Mum. I do a paper round so I've got some money for food.'
- 'Dad died 3 weeks ago. Mum's been drunk ever since. She threw me out tonight.'
- 'Dad's only like this because Mum died. He cries a lot and then goes to the pub. He only beats me after that.'

There is some evidence that school performance can be adversely affected in bereaved children (Barnardo's Orchard Project 1997) and potential links are being suggested between social exclusion and bereavement, youth offending, substance abuse, and teenage pregnancy (Sweeting *et al.* 1998), particularly when the death has been sudden and traumatic (Barnard *et al.* 1999; Boswell 2000). Dora Black summarizes the situation thus; 'Controlled studies based on population samples have confirmed earlier clinical impressions that bereaved children have a significantly increased risk of developing psychiatric disorders and may suffer considerable psychological and social difficulties throughout childhood and even later in adult life' (Black 1996). However, statistical evidence to highlight links between bereavement and social exclusion is scant and is not routinely collated. Research has not yet demonstrated exactly how and to what extent the various types of intervention offered to bereaved children may improve their life chances and capacity to manage grief, loss, and change. Despite growing evidence that bereaved children and families appreciate and benefit from access to a range of support, there is currently no consistent, pro-active system across the United Kingdom to ensure that all children and young people, together with their families and other caregivers, receive basic information, guidance, and support following a death in their family or community. For instance, there is no system to ensure that a school is informed when a child has been bereaved of a significant person in their lives. It is generally perceived to be the responsibility of the grieving family to inform the school of the bereavement and to negotiate support for the child from teachers and other staff, in the short and long term.

Little consistency exists in the provision of bereavement policies and support within schools throughout the United Kingdom. Much depends on the attitude of the head teachers and other senior staff, and their experience in dealing with death and bereavement issues. 'The first teacher I had was nice but the next teacher ..., she said – oh, it's over now, it's done. Whenever I went to talk to them, they just said sit back down' (Childhood Bereavement Network 2003*b*). In addition, there are no statutory requirements about general loss and death education in the curriculum.

One of the greatest challenges facing those who advocate for the rights of bereaved children and young people is how to raise the profile of childhood bereavement and to influence policy making at all levels. For example the United Kingdom Government Green Paper; 'Every Child Matters' (2003), does not include any reference to bereavement as a risk factor despite the paper's acknowledgement of the value of early intervention and family support to improve outcomes for 'at risk' children. Government rhetoric about 'joined up thinking and joined up services' has yet to be matched by coherent policy development. The CBN is campaigning with the National Children's Bureau to ensure that all government policy initiatives should acknowledge bereavement as a potential risk factor for children and young people, that everyone who works with, or has contact with children and young people, should receive mandatory bereavement awareness training and that statistical information and research in the area should be improved (CBN 2004).

Belief Statement

We believe that all children have the right to information, guidance and support to enable them to manage the impact of death on their lives.

Further, in line with the Children Act 1989 and the Children (Scotland) Act 1995, we believe that any information, guidance and support offered to children should:

- acknowledge the child's grief and experience of loss as a result of death

- be responsive to the child's needs, views and opinions

- respect the child's family and immediate social situation, and their culture, language, beliefs and religious background

- seek to promote self-esteem and self confidence, and develop communication, decision making and other life skills

- be viewed as part of a continuous learning process for the child, contributing to the development of the child's knowledge and understanding as they grow into adulthood

- aim, wherever possible, appropriate and feasible, to involve family members, other caregivers and any professionals working with the individual child in a wider social context.

If this information, guidance and support is offered as a service by an organisation or in a professional context, it should be:

- provided by people who have had appropriate training and who are adequately supported

- provided in an appropriately supportive, safe and non-discriminatory context

- regularly monitored, evaluated and reviewed.

Fig. 1.2 Childhood Bereavement Network Belief Statement.

Every child or young person will experience loss in some way. As adults, we cannot prevent and protect children from experiencing the pain of loss. However, bereaved children are entitled to feel secure and supported in the presence of caring adults; their carers, teachers, social workers, or doctors. Children have the right to expect that the caring professionals with whom they come into contact in the normal course of their lives, will be able to acknowledge their loss and understand the impact of that loss, at that moment and also into the future. Ironically, the needs of bereaved children are often very simple and immediate; a conversation or an opportunity to talk, to be heard and reassured, some practical advice and guidance and an acknowledgement of the loss.

The Belief Statement of the Childhood Bereavement Network (Fig. 1.2), which was developed in consultation with practitioners throughout the United Kingdom, provides policy guidance and promotes key principles for anyone working with or in contact with bereaved children, young people, and their families.

References

Barnard P, Morland I, Nagy J (1999). *Children, bereavement and trauma.* London: Jessica Kingsley.

Barnardo's Orchard Project and the City of Newcastle upon Tyne Education Service (1997). *Matters of life and death: a handbook of information and ideas for schools, children and parents about bereavement and loss.* Newcastle upon Tyne Local Education Authority, Newcastle.

Black D (1998). Coping with loss: bereavement in childhood. *BMJ* **316**: 931–3 (21 March).

Boswell G (2000). The backgrounds of violent young offenders, the present picture. In: G Boswell (ed.) *Violent children and adolescents.* London: Whurr Publishers.

Childhood Bereavement Network (2002). *Video: A death in the lives of…*

Childhood Bereavement Network (2003a). *Report on a mapping exercise to identify open access specialist bereavement support services for children and young people in England.*

Childhood Bereavement Network (2003b). *Video: You'll always remember them, even when you're old.*

Childhood Bereavement Network Policy Briefing (2004). London: National Children's Bureau.

Couldrick A (1988). *Grief and bereavement: understanding children.* Oxford: Sobell Publications.

Cross S (2002). *I can't stop feeling sad: calls to ChildLine about bereavement.* ChildLine Special Report: www.childline.org.uk

Department of Social Work, St Christopher's Hospice (1989). Someone special has died. London: St Christopher's Hospice.

Dyregrov A (1991). *Grief in children: a handbook for adults.* London: Jessica Kingsley.

Heegaard M (1998). *When someone very special dies.* Minneapolis, MN: Woodland Press.

Northampton Child & Family Consultation Service (1991). *Video. That morning I went to school.*

Pennells M, Smith S (1995). *Interventions with bereaved children.* London: Jessica Kingsley.

Rolls L, Payne S (2003). Childhood bereavement services: a survey of UK provision. *Palliative Medicine* 423–32.

Smith S, Pennells M (ed.) (1995). *Interventions with bereaved children.* London: Jessica Kingsley.

Stokes J (2004). *Then, now and always:* supporting children as they journey through grief-a practitioner's guide. Cheltenham: Winston's Wish.

Stokes J, Pennington J, Monroe B *et al.* (1999). Developing services for bereaved children: a discussion of the theoretical and practical issues involved. *Mortality* **4**(3):291–307

Sweeting H, West P, Richards M (1998). Teenage family life, lifestyles and life chances: associations with family structure, conflict with parents and joint family activity. *International Journal of Law, Policy and the Family* **12**, 15–46.

Treasury H M (2003). *Every child matters.* London: The Stationery Office.

Worden J W (1996). *Children and grief: when a parent dies.* New York: Guilford Press.

Chapter 2

Theoretical perspectives: linking research and practice

Ann Dent

Introduction

Every child is unique with a unique background. Children can experience death at any age from infancy to adulthood, during which time, each child is developing physically, emotionally, intellectually, spiritually, and socially. They may suffer the death of a parent, sibling, grandparent, or that of a close friend or family member. Death can be sudden and unexpected through accident, illness, suicide, murder, war, or natural disasters; or expected when death occurs from natural causes or a life-threatening disease. With so many variables, it is clear that childhood bereavement is a multi-faceted and complex subject. However, whatever the type of death, we now know that children grieve after a significant death, although they do so differently from adults (Corr and Corr 1996; Silverman 2000). Their 'reconstitution' is shaped by four factors: understanding the death, emotional reactions to the death, grieving and the reconstitution of the family (Christ 2000).

Although research into adult bereavement began nearly a century ago, it is only in recent years, in the Western world, that there has been a growing professional and public awareness of the needs of bereaved children. For instance, we now know that when the death of a parent is anticipated, children's bereavement may be affected by a number of factors, including the duration of the previous illness of the deceased parent (Black and Urbanowicz 1987), advance knowledge of the impending death and/or the degree of the child's awareness of their parent's death (Black and Urbanowicz 1987; Worden 1996). Such factors may affect a child's functioning before the death (Christ *et al.* 1993; Compas *et al.* 1994) and continue into the period immediately after the death (Christ 2000).

For children who experience sudden and unexpected death, there is no opportunity for preparation. Such deaths can be very distressing, especially when a body has been mutilated, or death was self-induced. Studies have consistently shown that subsequent adjustment can be more difficult, particularly immediately after the death (Furman 1983; Kranzler *et al.* 1990; Worden 1996).

Research into the death of a grandparent has been very limited, despite the fact that the bond between grandchildren and grandparents is 'second in emotional power and influence only to the relationship between parents and children' (cited in Renzenbrink 2002).

When a friend dies, children may be faced with the limitations of the way in which death is viewed in the wider world around them. The death may, or may not be acknowledged by the school and local community in the period immediately afterwards, but the long-term effects on a grieving child may not be fully recognized (Silverman 2000).

This chapter is an opportunity to explore various theories that have emerged from research. Most have been developed from research into bereaved adults; can they be adapted to fit the needs of bereaved children? I will consider the stage/phase theories, tasks of grief, the dual process model (DPM), and continuing bonds in relation to children's bereavement, using current research. The chapter begins by considering the development of children's conceptual thinking as a basis for understanding their concepts of death. As children do not live in isolation, the importance of family in shaping their responses and their subsequent bereavement will be discussed. The chapter will end by considering some of the research into different types of childhood bereavement, including the death of a parent, sibling, and grandparent.

Children's development of conceptual thinking

I am frequently asked in workshops for professionals at what age children understand death. This seems to be an important starting point for many. However, as Christ (2000) suggests, it is not so much the age of a child, but their cognitive developmental attributes, which provide essential information as to how a child thinks and processes such information.

Piaget (1954) identified four sequential phases in a child's development, through which thinking progresses: sensory-motor (infant), pre-operational (pre-school), concrete operational (school-age), and formal operational (adolescence). These stages reflect the changing perspectives from which children view the world and know others. Younger children who feel sad or frustrated are likely to cry, be demanding, and are unlikely to see the situation beyond its effect on them; whereas adolescents may have similar feelings but can put them into words and see the context that stimulated their feelings (Silverman 2000). As a child matures, his social world increases from the intimacy of the child/ home/parent, to interaction with family members, school, and friends, and eventually to a wider context where other factors such as the mass media and culture may influence them (Christ 2000).

Children's understanding of death

A mature view of death has been described as containing an understanding of the universality, irreversibility, non-functioning, and causality of death (Wass 1984; Speece and Brent 1996). In Kenyon's recent critical review of research into children's conceptions of death (2001), she concluded that most children understand death as a changed state by three years, by five or six understand that death is universal, although an understanding of what causes death comes slightly later. By 10 years, children are able to grasp universality, irreversibility, and personal mortality. However, their level of verbal ability, personal experience, the family's cultural and religious beliefs, and their environment are also important influencing factors. Much of the previous research was conducted with non-bereaved children, so Christ's work (2000) with 88 families and their 157 children, aged from three to 17 years, who coped with the terminal illness and consequent death of one of their parents, gives us valuable insights. Emerging from the data were five separate age groups, showing how cognitive, emotional, and social aspects of development shaped their responses (Christ 2000, pp. 38–39).

Age 3–5

Children of this age were unable to grasp the finality of their parent's death for several weeks or months. Separations from their primary caregiver gave rise to anxiety. They were unlikely to be affected by the world outside their family.

Age 6–8

These children understood the finality of the parent's death but often blamed themselves for the death. They could, with explanations, cope with separations of caregivers more easily than younger children. School life was beginning to widen their social understanding.

Age 9–11

These children had solid cognitive capacities, seeking detailed information about the illness and death, which gave them some control over the situation. They found grief hard to bear so school was a welcome escape. Support from adults, especially teachers, enhanced their self-esteem. Home, school, peers, and sports now affected their development. Other parents helped to enhance their 'reconstitution'.

Age 12–14

This was a transition period between late concrete and early operational capacities, giving rise to ambivalent dependence/independence.

Emotionally these young people withdrew from their parents, avoiding information, and others' grief reactions as well as their own. Activities outside the home took on more importance.

Age 15–17

These young people showed consistent operational capacities and had a more sophisticated understanding of future implications of the parent's illness and death. They were less dependent on caregivers than 12–14 year olds, seeking support from peers. Their grief was more like adults and they showed greater understanding of, and involvement with, their larger community.

Do children experience stages and phases of grief?

The first intra-psychic theory of grief was proposed by Freud (1917) and has stood as a precedent for scientific research into grief today. Lindemann's classic study of survivors of the Coconut Grove fire in Boston (1944) described adult grief as having both somatic and psychological effects, where distress, preoccupation with the deceased, guilt, anger, and loss of usual living pattern were experienced. Later Parkes, in the UK, as a result of his extensive work with widows (1972), described four phases of grief: numbness, pining, depression, and recovery.

In relation to bereaved children, Bowlby's work (1961) has great significance. He demonstrated that young children, separated from their mothers during World War II, grieved for the loss of a central figure, disturbing their sense of well-being. They experienced shock, numbness, disbelief, yearning, and searching, followed by despair and disorganization. Most were able to adjust to the new situation and develop new relationships. Bowlby emphasized the importance of a child's attachment to critical care-givers, and the impact that this had on their future development and adult life. Since Bowlby's seminal work, other researchers have found that bereaved children experience similar emotions to separated children (Furman 1974; Rosen 1986; Dyregrov 1991; Bluebond-Langner 1996; Worden 1996; Riches and Dawson 2000; Rosenblatt 2000; Silverman 2000). In Christ's study (2000), children of ages 3–5 experienced sad, unhappy, and angry feelings for many days or months; children of ages 6–8 initially cried and had temper tantrums, said and acted what they felt, and had increased anxiety about being separated from the surviving parent. Expressions of grief in those aged between nine and 11 tended to be subdued and their sadness did not have the overwhelming and helpless characteristics of younger children. Younger adolescents tended to keep their feelings to themselves but became angrier when pressures at school increased. Children of ages 15–17 years often experienced an initial period of numbness followed by an intense period of grieving. They experienced sustained bouts of profound sadness, crying, anger, bitterness, and depressed mood with sleep disturbances, and a sense of hopelessness or being overwhelmed.

The tasks of grief

By the 1980s, Worden viewed grief slightly differently. He conceived the grieving process in adults as an active experience where they can do much to help themselves by working through a series of tasks (1983, 1991). By 1996, Worden presented some of the major findings from the Harvard Child Bereavement Study, involving 70 families where a parent had died. From these families, 125 bereaved children were identified between the ages of six and 17 and matched with non-bereaved children by age, gender, grade in school, family religion, and community. Semi-structured interviews with children and their surviving parent were conducted at four months from the death and soon after the first and second anniversaries.

As a result of his findings, Worden suggested that his 'tasks' for adults also apply to children 'but can only be understood in terms of the cognitive, emotional and social development of the child' (Worden 1996, p. 2).

According to Worden (1996, p. 13–16), these tasks are:

To accept the reality of the loss

Initially children need to be told of the death accurately and in age-appropriate language. This may need to be given repeatedly, especially for younger children, and when the death is sudden. Children have as great a need as adults to make the unreal real and to gain a concrete basis for their grief rather than fantasies. After careful explanation, being given the opportunity to see a dead body and attending the funeral may help a child to accept the reality of death more easily (Dyregrov 1991). Christ (2000) found that most children in her study under five years had attended the funeral, and although they did not understand the symbolism, they clearly gained from participation.

To experience the pain and emotional aspects of the loss

Bereaved children experience a wide range of feelings, which need to be acknowledged and worked through gradually, so that they are not overwhelmed. Children between six and eight years are particularly vulnerable, as they understand something about the permanence of death but have yet to develop the social skills to deal with any intensity of feelings (Christ 2000). Much will depend on how the surviving parent and others deal with their feelings. Ambivalent relationships with the deceased may cause children to feel angry or regretful. Children of nine to 11 years have the capacity for logical thinking, but have a tendency to subdue intense emotional reactions (Christ 2000). Doing things together as a family and sharing memories of the dead parent, may encourage children to grieve (Christ 2000).

To adjust to an environment in which the deceased is missing

Much will depend on the role and relationship the child had with the deceased parent and also in the life of the family. Worden (1996) found that the death of a mother results in more daily life changes than the death of a father. The more the changes, the greater the need for adjustment. Although a child may 'get over' the death, grief may surface years later at special times, such as getting a job, graduating from University, getting married, or having a baby. The 'cascade' of events described by Christ (2000) suggests that as children go through different developmental stages, varying stressful events may have a cumulative effect. These may affect children's self-esteem or confidence, influencing their perception and/or responses to subsequent events.

To relocate the dead person and find ways to memorialize the person

The death of a parent is permanent, but the process of loss continues, as part of a child's ongoing experience. The main aim of this task is to enable a child to find a new and appropriate place for the dead parent so that they can go on to live effectively. How do they view this now-dead parent? Are they able to put the relationship in a new context rather than severing all ties?

The dual process model: a suitable model for bereaved children?

A recent and significant advance in our understanding of grief is the dual process model (DPM) developed by Stroebe and Schut (1999). Through extensive research with bereaved adults (Stroebe 1992), they concluded that grief is a dynamic process in which there is oscillation between focusing on (loss-orientation) and avoiding the loss (restoration-orientation). Loss-orientation encompasses grief work and restoration-orientation includes dealing with secondary losses as a result of the death, such as coping with everyday life, building a new identity, and seeking distraction from painful thoughts. By taking time off from the pain of grief, which may overwhelm them, the bereaved may be more able to cope with daily life and the secondary changes that death brings.

As the DPM was developed with adults in mind, is it applicable to bereaved children? When a significant death occurs in a child's life, (s)he too will be grieving for the deceased but may also have to cope with secondary losses, arising from the death. A child whose parent dies is likely to experience a time of family disruption, causing anxiety and confusion (Christ 2000; Silverman 2000). The surviving parent's distress may be alien to a child, resulting in feelings of powerlessness at how to make things better. Lack of discipline and any structured routine is likely to cause further confusion and anxiety. Christ (2000) found that children worried about who would comb their hair, take care of them when they were sick, help them with their homework.

The death of a sibling will cause grief over the dead child but will also bring changes to the world in which the siblings live (Silverman 2000).

Children also need time away from the constant pain of grief. Children of school age spend a large part of their week in school. Being busy with other things can be helpful, just as it can help adults who return to work. It may be a diversion and a place where they are not constantly reminded of the death, a time to take a break from the grieving family (Silverman 2000).

Continuing bonds

Commenting on the work of Bowlby (1980) and Raphael (1984), Walter (1996, p. 7) made the following remark: 'This body of work has been widely read to say that the purpose of grief is the reconstitution of an autonomous individual who can in large measure leave the deceased behind and form new attachments.' In practice, this has been taken to imply that ending the relationship with the deceased is required, in other words 'breaking bonds'. However, recently this has been questioned. Instead of 'letting go', is it possible to have an on-going presence of the deceased so that a connection or relationship continues?

In *Continuing Bonds: New Understandings of Grief* (Klass *et al.* (eds.) 1996), different contributors maintain that the resolution of grief involves continuing bonds with the deceased and that such bonds are a healthy part of on-going life. In one chapter, Silverman and Nickman (1996) discuss their findings from a longitudinal prospective study, where children aged from 6 to 17 years and their surviving parents were interviewed.

Analysis revealed that children talked about their dead parent maintaining relationships, rather than letting go. The children had sets of memories, feelings and behaviours, which they maintained, brought them closer to their dead parents, so that the children remained in relationship with them. As the children grew up and the intensity of their grief lessened, the relationship changed. Rather than 'resolving grief' it appeared to comfort children and assisted them with their grief. Christ (2000) found that up to the age of 12, most children enjoyed focusing on memories, dreamt and conversed with their dead parent. They valued tokens of remembrance such as photographs, jewellery, and clothing. Children aged 12–14 years found that thinking or talking of their dead parent interfered with their main preoccupation of school and peers. In an effort to control emotions, any reminders were difficult for them. However, they valued something belonging to the dead parent and tried to maintain contact through activities that reminded them of the dead parent. Older adolescents continued to internalize the past relationship with the dead parent, wanting to be alone, so that they could think of the dead parent and grieve in their own way. They were keen to do what the parent had expected of them and to live up to those expectations. In relation to bereaved sibling adolescents, Hogan and Desantis (1992) found that 'ongoing attachment' (emotional and social) continues throughout the bereavement process. As Silverman and Nickman suggest:

> Learning to remember and finding a way of maintaining a connection to the deceased, consistent with the child's cognitive development and family dynamics, are also normative aspects of the accommodation process that allows children to go on living in the face of loss.
> (Silverman and Nickman 2000, p. 74)

Thus children can continue to have a connection as part of a functional adaptation, where the dead parent or sibling is remembered and may remain as a guide and witness for continued living.

Bereaved children experience a range of feelings, and it is likely that the tasks of grief, originally developed for adults, are also applicable to children. Bereaved children can also oscillate between loss-orientation and restoration-orientation, so that the DPM is a suitable model. Children, like adults, need to maintain bonds with the deceased, and therefore the notion of continuing bonds for children is very relevant.

The importance of family

It is impossible to talk about children without including the family (Silverman 2000). Most children grow up in their biological families where parents influence their feelings, attitudes, and behaviour. For others, such as foster children, the adults around them play a significant part in their development. From an early age, children begin to learn about loss and how to deal with it (Viorst 1989). Children are weaned, and go to nursery school, where they leave their parents for a short time. The birth of a new baby may temporarily (or permanently) disrupt their security within the family. As they grow older they go to school for longer periods, may move house, losing friends and familiarity, or cope with the death of a pet. The manner in which parents deal with these early losses may stand as a precedent for more major losses, such as the death of a parent or sibling (Silverman 2000). It is also important to recognize that growth is a two-way process. Children can also make contributions to the family by stimulating responses in the adults around them, and influencing them (Bell and Harper 1977).

Every family is unique; each makes its own boundaries, develops ways of communicating (or not), constructs ways of making meaning that reflects who its members are, and develops problem-solving strategies and styles of coping in a crisis. The family's flexibility and openness to new ideas are important factors in how its members behave in any new situation (Reiss 1981; Olsen *et al.* 1989). Thus when a significant death occurs, the ways in which the family as a whole deals with it, may be reflected in how other losses have been dealt with.

Grief has been described as a family developmental crisis, interwoven with the family's history and its current development, where the family's grief redirects their future life together (Shapiro 1996). As Rosenblatt suggests:

> Individual grief is often profoundly shaped by the family context in which it occurs and often has profound affects on the bereaved person's family. Day to day life in any family— family routines, communication, shared realities, times of anger and disappointment, and so on—may be strongly influenced by bereavement, even for losses of decades ago .
> (Rosenblatt 2002, p. 125).

Moos (1995) suggests that each family member has to be open with the others if they are to share feelings about a death and about how the family needs to change. When this is not possible, then the whole family system is affected, as how each family member copes with the death, will be influenced by the others. When grief reactions, whether those of a child or adult, are ignored, discouraged or produce unbearable distress in others, opportunities to reminisce about the deceased are reduced (Riches and Dawson 2000).

A significant death may change family roles. Each member's needs may be different, with confusion and disagreement resulting as each seeks their own solution (Riches and Dawson 2000). A death can trigger painful differences in how each makes meaning of it and deals with it.

Families making meaning of the death

Nadeau's work (1998) has provided interesting insights into 'family meaning-making'. She identified factors that inhibited and enhanced the process.

Enhancers include frequency of family contact, rituals, and a willingness of family members to share meaning. Inhibitors include fragile family relationships, secrets, and divergent beliefs of family members. Although her work with families did not include children, her findings could equally apply to families with children.

As Middleton and Edwards posit (1990), effective mourning requires someone to mourn to, so that conversation is crucial to a family's attempt to make sense of the death. Although Walter is referring to adults, talking about the dead person may be equally important to children. He suggests: 'Survivors typically want to talk about the deceased and to talk with others who knew him or her. Together they construct a story that places the dead within their lives, a story capable of enduring through time' (Walter, 1996, p. 7).

Frank (1995, p. 53) proposed that stories offer a 'way of drawing maps and finding new destinations' for one's own identity. No matter how young children are, they struggle too to make sense of what is happening (Rogoff 1994). Children are not passive participants in the life of the family but will actively make meaning out of their experiences. The meaning they make will depend on their age, stage of development, and experience in life (Silverman 2000), and is also influenced by other family members.

The death of a parent

The death of a parent leads to a radical change in a child's life (Silverman 2000). The degree of openness of family communication prior to the death (Silverman 2000; Christ 2000) and the flexibility of families in facing the new reality, are both issues to consider. Whatever the age, Worden (1996) suggests that the functional level of the surviving parent is the most powerful predictor of a child's adjustment. The quality of care of the child and the child's relationship with the surviving parent have been identified consistently as affecting the course and outcome of a child's bereavement (Breier et al. 1988; Sood et al. 1992; Worden 1996; Lutzke et al. 1997; Christ 2000; Silverman 2000). Parents who are less depressed and cope actively after the death, are more likely to contribute to a child's better functioning (Kranzler et al. 1990; Worden 1996), as are the parent's warmth and family cohesion (Bifulco et al. 1987; Strength 1991; Lutzke et al. 1997; Christ 2000). Bereaved children are more likely to experience anxiety, depression, as well as sleep and health problems when a parent is functioning less well, although having the support of a number of siblings can mitigate against this (Worden 1996).

In comparing younger and older children bereaved of a parent, Worden (1996) found that children aged between 6 and 11 years appeared to be more affected by the behaviour of their peers, experienced more social difficulties in the second year, cried more frequently and had more health problems soon after the death which, in some cases, continued into the second year.

Sudden death of a parent is likely to lead to worse adaptation at one year, and when there are concurrent family stresses, children are likely to have more behavioural changes (Worden 1996). Mother-loss causes more dramatic emotional/behavioural disturbances than father-loss, such as higher levels of anxiety, more acting-out, lower self-esteem, and less belief in self-efficacy (Worden 1996; Silverman 2000). In some families, a child's adaptation may be hindered not so much by the death itself, but by a series or cascade of other stresses, related or unrelated to the death (Christ 2000). As a parent's death may have different meanings for each in a family, it is also not unusual for one child to adapt well, and another to have delayed or compromised grief (Christ, 2000).

Two important factors arose from the narratives of Christ's study (2000): firstly that surviving parents can grieve deeply but can still be available, support and enable their children to continue with the tasks of ongoing development. Secondly, there is no one right way to grieve and reach 'reconstitution'.

The death of a sibling

The sibling relationship is unique and likely to be the longest social connection made by individuals (Rando 1989). Siblings share a range of experiences and activities, confide in each other, and/or challenge parental authority (Martinson and Campos 1991). On the other hand, each has a unique experience in the family, dependent on age, birth order, and the relationships with their parents and other siblings (Dunn and Plomin 1990). Thus, the death of a sibling has consequences for self-identity, relationships with parents and other surviving siblings, as well as for long-term relationships in adult life (Lewis and Schonfield 1994; Robinson and Mahon 1997).

Recent research in the U.S. (summarized in Davies 1999) reveals some important findings. Bereaved siblings were found to have lower social competence (Birenbaum 1990), social withdrawal, and feelings of 'being different' from other children (Davies 1991). Adolescents experienced more anxiety, guilt, and depression than younger children (Fanos 1991). Children of ages 4 to 11 had increased behavioural problems (Hutton 1994; McCown and Davies 1995) and were more likely to be stubborn, irritable, and argumentative. Two recent UK studies (Dent *et al.* 1996; Dent 2000) revealed that behaviour changes in bereaved siblings were common. Parents bereaved of a child, reported that the majority of their surviving children ($N = 150$, aged from 10 months to 15 years) had experienced behavioural changes from six months to two years, after the death of their sibling. Aggression appeared to be the commonest change, especially in the first six months. Becoming withdrawn, bed-wetting, being 'clingy', telling lies, being bullied, and being unable to concentrate were also reported.

However, as Heiney points out (1991), negative consequences are not inevitable. It is how the family as a whole copes with a child's death that determines the quality of the surviving siblings' adjustment. Bereaved siblings' grief appears to be expressed more openly if they perceive their social networks as loving, respectful, and caring towards them (Hogan and Desantis 1992, 1994). Several researchers suggest that it is not so much the death that causes difficulties but the family system, which ultimately determines the long-term effects on siblings (Bradach and Jordan 1995; Black 1996; Rubin 1996). Sadly, Riches and Dawson (2000) found that many bereaved siblings of all ages expressed feelings of being left out, ignored, and isolated within the family.

Comparing sibling and parental loss

Although few studies have compared sibling and parent loss, Worden compared his findings from the Harvard Bereavement Study on death of a parent (Worden 1996), with several studies on sibling bereavement (Davies 1987, 1988a, b, 1991; McCown 1987; McCown and Pratt 1985). He found that there were few differences. He suggests that the death of a parent produces no more emotional or behavioural difficulties than the death of a sibling during the first year of bereavement, with a quarter of children being 'at risk', regardless of type of death during the first six months. He further suggests that family influences that place children at risk, are equally likely for both types of death. These risks include: a larger number of children in the family, higher levels of concurrent family stresses, inadequate support from family and others, and passive coping styles of the parent(s).

However, in comparing gender, he noted that in general, boys were more affected by the death of a parent than by the death of a sibling. Pre-adolescent boys whose parent had died were more withdrawn, anxious, depressed, and exhibited more somatic problems than those who had lost a sibling. Both pre-adolescent and adolescent boys who had experienced the death of a parent were likely to be more in the 'at risk' group than those who had lost a sibling.

On the other hand, girls were more affected by the death of a sibling, especially adolescents who showed disturbed behaviour, higher levels of anxiety, depression, and attention-seeking behaviours than those who had been bereaved of a parent. Pre-adolescent and adolescent girls bereaved of a sibling were more likely to be 'at risk' than those whose parent had died.

The death of a grandparent

As stated earlier, little research has been conducted into the death of a grandparent although this must be one of the commonest deaths that children face (Renzenbrink 2002). However, two studies carried out by Irizzary in Australia (1988) give valuable insights. The first involved 56 children (30 girls and 26 boys) predominantly Anglo-Australian and Christian, aged eight to 13 years. The second was a cross-cultural comparison and replication of the first involving 12 girls and nine boys, mostly from a European and Jewish background. Using semi-structured interviews, Irizzary found some differences between the groups, the children reporting vivid and detailed recollections of the events surrounding their grandparents' deaths. Many of the children had wanted more information, and felt that their parents were holding back, but did not ask for fear of upsetting them. Sadness and regret were common due to being unable to do previous activities with the dead grandparent.

In conclusion, Irizzary reported that children's responses were very similar to those of adults in terms of depth of emotion, vividness of recall, the quality of descriptions, and the longing for things to be different. Many children felt excluded from rituals and decisions about the form they should take. The children also demonstrated that they maintained connection with the dead grandparent in memory, thought, and actions. Because some children remained quiet about their feelings, parents were unaware of the depth, curiosities, worries, and impressions that their children experienced.

Summary

Children's understanding of death concepts develops gradually, but by around nine to ten years most will have grasped that it is inevitable, irreversible, and universal. Whilst age is one predictor, it is also influenced by children's cognitive, emotional, and social development, by past death experiences, verbal ability, and the attitudes of others around them.

The bereavement theories, initially developed from research into bereaved adults, would also appear relevant for bereaved children. Children experience loss feelings similar to bereaved adults, and may need help in working through the tasks suggested by Worden. Children also oscillate between adjusting to their changed environment, grieving for the dead person and needing time away from the pain. Children, like adults, do not have to 'break bonds' with the deceased but need continuing bonds, which may bring comfort to guide them in their future life.

The family plays a significant part in the life of any bereaved child. How children of all ages experience and respond to death, will be reflected in what they have learnt and experienced previously. It is within the family that we begin to understand how different people cope with death. Children need opportunities to talk about their feelings and to make some sense of them and the death in a confusing new world. Bereaved siblings particularly tend to be ignored and isolated within their family. Throughout the literature, the importance of how the parent(s) cope with the death, whether of a parent, sibling, or grandparent is constantly reinforced.

References

Bell RQ, Harper L (1977). *Child effects on adults*. Hillsdale, NJ: Lawrence Erlbaum Associates.

Bifulco A, Brown G, Harris T (1987). Childhood loss of a parent, lack of adequate parental care and adult depression: a replication. *Social Psychology* **16**:187–97.

Birenbaum LK, Robinson MA, Phillips DS *et al.* (1990). The response of children to the dying and death of a sibling. *Omega* **20**:213–28.

Black D (1996). Childhood bereavement. *British Medical Journal* **312**(7045):1496.

Black D, Urbanowicz M (1987) Family interventions with bereaved children. *Journal of Psychology and Psychiatry* **28**:467–76.

Bowlby J (1961). Processes of mourning. *International Journal of Psycho-Analysis* **42**(4–5):317–39.

Bowlby J (1980). *Attachment and loss*, Vol 3, 1st edn. New York: Basic Books.

Bradach KM, Jordan JR (1995). Long term effects of a family history of traumatic death on adolescent individuation. *Death Studies* **19**(4):315–36.

Breier A, Kelso J, Kirwin P (1988). Early parental loss and development of adult psychopathology. *Archives of General Psychiatry* **45**:987–93.

Compas B, Worsham N, Epping-Jordan J *et al.* (1994). When mom or dad has cancer: Markers of psychological distress in cancer patients, spouses and children. *Health Psychology* **13**:507–15.

Christ G (2000). *Healing children's grief: surviving a parent's death from cancer*. Oxford: Oxford University Press.

Christ G, Siegal K, Freund B *et al.* (1993). Impact of parental terminal cancer on latency-age children. *American Journal of Orthopsychiatry* **61**:417–25.

Corr C, Corr D (1996). *Handbook of childhood death and bereavement*. New York: Springer.

Davies B (1987). Family responses to the death of a child: The meaning of memories. *Journal of Palliative Care* **3**:9–15.

Davies B (1988*a*). Shared life space and sibling bereavement responses. *Cancer Nursing* **11**:339–47.

Davies B (1988*b*). The family environment in bereaved families and its relationship to surviving sibling behaviour. *Child Health Care* **17**:22–32.

Davies B (1991). Long-term outcomes of adolescent sibling bereavement. *Journal of Adolescent Research* **6**:83–96.

Davies B (1999). *Shadows in the sun: the experiences of sibling bereavement in childhood.* London: Brunner/Mazel.

Dent A (2000). Support for families whose child dies suddenly from accident or illness. Doctoral thesis, School of Policy Studies, University of Bristol.

Dent A, Condon L, Fleming P *et al.* (1996). A study of bereavement care after sudden and unexpected death. *Archives of Disease in Childhood* **74**(6):522–6.

Dunn J, Plomin R (1990). *Separate lives: why siblings are different.* New York: Basic Books.

Dyregrov A (1991). *Grief in children: a handbook for adults.* London: Jessica Kingsley.

Fanos JH, Nickerson BG (1991). Long-term effects of sibling death during adolescence. *Journal of Adolescent Research* **6**:70–82.

Frank A (1995). *The wounded storyteller.* Chicago: University of Chicago Press.

Freud S (1917) Mourning and melancholia. In: J Strachey (ed. and trans.), *Standard edition of the complete psychological works of Sigmund Freud.* London: Hogarth Press (1957).

Furman E (1974). A child's parent dies: studies in childhood bereavement. New Haven, CT: Yale University Press.

Furman E (1983). Studies in childhood bereavement. *Canadian Journal of Psychiatry* **28**:241–7.

Heiney SP (1991). Sibling grief: a case report. *Archives of Psychiatric Nursing* **5**(3):121–7.

Hogan N, DeSantis L (1994). Things that help and hinder adolescent sibling bereavement. *Western Journal of Nursing Research* **16**(2):132–53.

Hogan N, DeSantis L (1992). Adolescent sibling bereavement: an ongoing attachment. *Qualitative Health Research* **2**(2):159–77.

Hutton CJ, Bradley BS (1994). Effects of sudden infant death on bereaved siblings: a comparative study. *Journal of Child Psychology and Psychiatry* **35**:723–32.

Izzary C (1988). Childhood bereavement reactions to the death of a grandparent. Unpublished PhD thesis, Rutgers University, New Jersey.

Kenyon B (2001). Current research in children's conceptions of death: a critical review. *OMEGA, Journal of Death and Dying* **43**(1):63–91.

Klass D, Silverman S, Nickman S (ed.) (1996). *Continuing bonds. New understandings of grief.* Washington, DC: Taylor & Francis.

Kranzler E, Shaffer D, Wasserman G *et al.* (1990). Early childhood bereavement. *Journal of the American Academy of Child/Adolescent Psychiatry* **29**:513–20.

Lewis M, Schonfield D (1994). Role of child and adolescent psychiatric consultation and liaison in assisting children and their families in dealing with death. *Child and Adolescent Psychiatric Clinics of North America* **3**(3):613–27.

Lindemann E (1944). Symptomatology and management of acute grief. *American Journal of Psychiatry* **101**(Sept):141–8.

McCown D (1987). Factors related to children's behavioural adjustment. In: C Barnes (ed.) *Recent advances in nursing,* pp. 89–93. London: Churchill Livingstone.

McCown D, Pratt C (1985). Impact of sibling bereavement on children's behaviour. *Death Studies* **9**:323–35.

McCown DE, Davies B (1995). Patterns of grief in young children following the death of a sibling. *Death Studies* **19**:41–53.

Martinson I, Campos RG (1991). Adolescent bereavement: long-term responses to a sibling's death from cancer. *Journal of Adolescent Research* 6(1):54–69.

Middleton D, Edwards D (1990). Conversational remembering: a social-psychological approach. In: D Edwards, D Middleton (ed.) *Collective remembering.* London: Sage.

Moos N (1995). An integrative model of grief. *Death Studies* 19(4):337–64.

Nadeau J (1998). Families making sense of death. Thousand Oaks, CA: Sage.

Olsen DH, McCubbin HI, Barnes HL *et al.* (1989). *Families, what makes them work?* Newbury Park, CA: Sage.

Parkes C (1972). *Bereavement: studies in grief in adult life.* London: Tavistock.

Piaget J (1954). *The construction of reality in the child.* New York: Basic Books.

Rando T (1989). Parental adjustment to the loss of a child. In: D Papadatou, C Papadatos (ed.) *Children and death* pp. 233–53. New York: Hemisphere Publishing Corporation.

Raphael B (1984). *The anatomy of bereavement,* 3rd edn. London: Unwin Hyman.

Reiss D (1981). *The family's construction of reality.* Cambridge, MA: Harvard University Press.

Renzenbrink I (2002). In my heart he's still there: children's responses to the death of a grandparent. *Bereavement Care* 21(1):6–8.

Riches G, Dawson P (2000). *An intimate loneliness: supporting bereaved parents and siblings.* Buckingham, UK: Open University Press.

Rosen H (1986). *Unspoken grief: coping with childhood sibling loss.* Toronto: Lexington Books.

Rosenblatt P (2002). Guest editorial: Grief in families. *Mortality* 7(2):125–6.

Rogoff B (1994). Cross-cultural perspectives on children's development. In: PK Bock (ed.) *Psychological anthropology,* pp. 231–42. Westport, CT: Praeger.

Rubin SS (1996). The wounded family: bereaved parents and the impact of adult child loss. In: D Klass, P Silverman, S Nickman (ed.) *Continuing bonds: new understandings of grief.* Washington, DC: Taylor and Francis.

Segal NL, Wilson SM, Bouchard TJ *et al.* (1995). Comparative grief experiences of bereaved twins and other bereaved relatives. *Personality and individual differences* 18(4):511–24.

Shapiro E (1996). Family bereavement and cultural diversity: a social developmental perspective. *Family Process* 35(Sept):313–32.

Silverman P (2000). *Never too young to know.* New York: Oxford University Press.

Silverman P, Nickman S (1996). *Concluding thoughts.* In: D Klass, P Silverman, S Nickman (ed.) *Continuing bonds. New understandings of grief,* pp. 349–55. Philadelphia: Taylor and Francis.

Sood B, Weller K, Fristad M *et al.* (1992). Somatic complaints in grieving children. *Comprehensive Mental Care* 2:17–25.

Speece MW, Brent SB (1996). The development of the concept of death among Chinese and U.S. children 3–17 years of age: From binary to fuzzy concepts? *OMEGA* 33:67–83.

Strength J (1991). Factors influencing the mother-child relationship following the death of the father and how the relationship affects the child's functioning. Unpublished doctoral dissertation, Rosemead School of Psychology, La Mirada, CA.

Stroebe MS (1992–3). Coping with bereavement: a review of the grief work hypothesis. *OMEGA, Journal of Death and Dying* 26(1):19–42.

Stroebe M, Schut H (1999). The dual process model of coping with bereavement: rationale and description. *Death Studies* 23(3):197–224.

Viorst J (1989). *Necessary losses.* London: Positive Paperbacks.

Wass H (1984). Concepts of death: a developmental perspective. In: H Wass, C Corr (ed.) *Childhood and death,* pp. 3–24. Washington DC: Hemisphere.

Walter T (1996). A new model of grief: bereavement and biography. *Mortality* **1**(1):7–27.

Worden JW (1983). *Grief counselling and grief therapy,* 1st edn. London: Tavistock.

Worden JW (1991). *Grief counselling and grief therapy,* 2nd edn. London: Routledge.

Worden JW (1996). *Children and grief: when a parent dies.* New York: Guilford Press.

Chapter 3

Family assessment[1]

Julie Stokes

How families experience bereavement

'The family' is often a key context for determining the development and well-being of children who grow up within a family. As such, the family is a crucial component of any assessment of a bereaved child or young person who may be in need of a bereavement service. The assessment also needs to extend to other key relationships and contexts, for example, school, peers, and so on. Each family is different. Everyone will experience their grief differently: this will be shaped by their individual, family, cultural, social, and religious beliefs, and means that no two deaths are ever mourned in exactly the same way.

During the early weeks and months after a death, the family unit is inevitably fragile, vulnerable, and seemingly frozen in time. Shapiro (1994) describes grief as a crisis which becomes interwoven with family history, and has a dramatic effect on how the family develops as a new unit—'a family in developmental crisis'. Each family will struggle to stabilize after a death, and its first priority in managing the crisis is to work towards a stable equilibrium within which the family can try to move forward. 'With a developmental approach that considers the family as a unit of distinct yet inextricably interconnected members, we can help families survive and grow while bearing the burden of death and loss' (Shapiro 1994).

Assessing the family as a whole provides insight into the way a child is related to as part of a family group. This information is central to understanding the ways in which a family is able to safeguard and promote the well-being of the child, and whether there are aspects of family life and relationships which compromise its capacity to do so.

A family assessment provides a vehicle for observing and describing what the practitioner can learn from talking with families and from their interaction together. The technique used can be a positive intervention in itself; promoting clarity and understanding of how individuals within a family are experiencing the bereavement. It is a way of learning about families in a detailed, relatively objective, evidence-based

[1] Adapted from 'Preparing for the journey'. pp. 48–67 (Stokes JA (2004). In *Then, now and always: supporting children as they journey through grief-a guide for practitioners.* Cheltenham: Winston's Wish).

profile of family competence, considering family strengths alongside difficulties (Glaser *et al.* 1984).

Although this chapter will focus on the process of conducting an assessment in the family home, the same principles apply for a telephone or an outpatient assessment.

Aims of the assessment

The assessment aims to establish:

- the impact of this particular death
- for this particular family
- at this particular time
- living in this particular community.

In making the assessment, the key determinants of grief identified by Parkes and Weiss (1983) need to be considered (see Table 3.1).

Table 3.1 Determinants of grief

1. Who the person was in relation to them	To know about a person's grief response we need to know who the deceased was. This is a very simple, but powerful determinant of grief. Was the person who died a spouse or a child? A friend or a neighbour? For example, grief after the death of a child is likely to be expressed differently to grief following the death of a grandparent.
2. The nature of the attachment	The nature of the attachment between the person who died, and the griever is also important to the grief reaction displayed, and this is influenced by aspects outlined below.
a) Strength of the attachment	The strength of the attachment between the griever and the deceased underlines the grief response. An increased intensity of attachment tends to be associated with greater intensity of grief.
b) Security of the attachment	The sense of security provided from the attachment also contributes to the grief response. Did the existence of the deceased provide security in the griever's life? If so, this may exacerbate their grief response. Did the deceased boost the griever's self-esteem? If so, following the death of this important person, their self-esteem may be adversely affected and increase the intensity of their grief response.
c) Ambivalence of the relationship	The extent of ambivalence within a relationship is a very important grief determinant. What was the proportion of positive and negative feelings involved in the relationship? If the relationship was highly ambivalent and negative feelings were almost experienced in equal amounts to positive feelings, the grief may be expressed extremely intensely and in a difficult manner often involving anger and guilt.
d) Conflicts with the deceased	Conflicts with the deceased throughout life can influence the grief reaction and guilt involved. This can range from the normal, everyday relationship conflicts to physical and sexual abuse (Krupp *et al.* 1986).

Table 3.1 cont'd

3. Mode of death	How the person died also contributes to the grief response. Modes of death are typically categorized as: natural, accidental, suicidal and homicidal (NASH). Grief responses will manifest differently according to the mode of death. Other factors important to the grief response are the location of the death, whether the death was sudden or to some extent expected, and the situation in which the death occurred. For example, did the griever have any involvement in the accident in which the person died? This would have a profound effect on the grief response, possibly involving feelings of guilt.
4. Historical antecedents	Any losses the griever has had prior to the death (for example, illness, divorce, other deaths, redundancy), how these were dealt with and the outcome of these losses are important to the grief reaction displayed. More specifically, how the individual cognitively views these losses and adversities within their life is important. For example, a history of mental illness or even the death of another loved one would play a central role in the grief response.
5. Personality variables	Personality variables of the griever play significant role in the grief response. Bowlby's (1980) instrumental work on attachment and loss has been the main advocate for taking personality variables into account in the case of grief reactions. These factors include age, sex, openness with feelings, how they cope with anxiety, how they cope with stress in general, dependence on others and ease/difficulty of forming relationships. The grief reaction may be exacerbated in those who suffer from any 'personality disorder'.
6. Social variables	Social variables can be very important determinants of how an individual displays their grief reaction: social, ethnic, and religious factors will all play a role in forming this background for an individual. Religious and cultural backgrounds determine practice of rituals following a death and influence the mode and extent that grief is expressed. The level of perceived social support from others can also influence the intensity of the grief reaction.
7. Rituals	Participation in death-related rituals and activities: was there a ritual or not? If so, how did the grieving person participate and how was such participation experienced, what kind of involvement did the person have in decisions regarding the commemoration of the deceased, the handling of his or her belongings and so on?
8. Concurrent stressors	Additional life stressors following the death can make the grief even more intense. For example, the development of financial worries as a result of a decline in household income since a partner's death may increase the intensity of grief.

Adapted from Parkes and Weiss (1983) in Worden (1996)

The purpose of the home assessment is to:

◆ build trust so that the family feels 'safe' working with the organization/counsellor

◆ give information about the possible interventions so that the family can make an informed decision about future involvement

◆ collect information about the person who has died and attempt to understand how the death has affected the child(ren), other members of the family, and the wider community

◆ find out about the child's knowledge and understanding of death

◆ demonstrate how we can safely talk to children about death and grief

◆ allow the family to talk about the death in as much detail as they want to: this can be the first opportunity they have had to do this, and is often a therapeutic intervention for the family

◆ evaluate the degree of resilience/vulnerability observed in the family

◆ assess whether the services on offer could enhance resilience/reduce vulnerability

◆ assess whether referral onto another agency is also appropriate

◆ draw up an action plan: this may include some time to think and reflect before deciding to participate in the suggested intervention.

Who is involved in the assessment?

At Winston's Wish (a community child bereavement programme) it is our usual practice for two practitioners to make the initial visit; this helps to ensure that each family member has a chance to share their story individually. It also enables the practitioners to be confident that they themselves have reached a shared understanding of the key issues relevant for this particular family.

The following case study summarizes some key issues that emerged from a home assessment of an adolescent boy and his grandmother.

Case Study: Ben (14)

A referral was received from Ben's head teacher. Ben has been having significant problems at school and was currently excluded following a mobile phone theft and abusive behaviour. His mother died 3 years ago in a car accident and he now lives with his maternal grandmother.

A phone call to his grandmother (Anne) gathers additional information; Ben has a stepsister (Jemma) aged 8. Ben had lived with his mother and his step-father until his mother's death. Since then Ben has experienced a difficult relationship with his step-father who was driving the car at the time his mother died. Given the tense family dynamics it is negotiated that the first assessment involved meeting with Ben and Anne at home with a view to making contact with Ben's step family (if appropriate) after that initial meeting.

A home assessment was arranged. Ben met with a practitioner on his own and his grand-mother also had an opportunity to share her story with another practitioner. At the end everyone met up to discuss the best way forward. The assessment revealed that Ben harbours some strong feelings of regret and resentment over his mother's death. He explained that he had planned to join them on the car trip but refused to go shopping at the last minute and stayed with a neighbour playing computer games.

It transpires that Ben believes his step-father was driving dangerously and that the accident would not have happened if he had been there. The accident happened at the beginning of the school holidays and it resulted in Ben moving out of his family home to live with Anne and a change to his planned secondary school move. He moved 10 miles away and lost regular contact with friends and his sister. He said his grandmother had threatened to put him in a home if his behaviour didn't improve. He admitted to stealing money to buy drugs to escape from it all.

The assessment identified a number of issues which would be addressed during a series of six individual sessions using a cognitive behavioural approach. The service also looked at facilitating links with his step-father and sister with a view to enabling the family to attend a residential weekend group intervention. Ben also gave his permission for the assessment report to be sent to his year tutor, so the school had a clearer understanding of the issues he was facing following his mother's death.

Skills needed by practitioners

The ability to understand the influence of a variety of interconnecting factors is an essential skill in carrying out a systemic assessment. Grief is a deeply shared family developmental transition, involving a crisis of attachment and a crisis of identity for family members, both of which have to be incorporated into the on-going flow of family development. The assessment process needs to take stock of all facets of the family system both before and after the development has been interrupted by death and grief. A structured assessment pack is used to ensure a systemic framework is adopted for all assessments. However, experienced practitioners will inevitably use their 'clinical intuition' to decide the order of questions rather than rigidly following the order of questions in the pack. Such clinical intuition makes sure they engage with family members and allows individuals to work in their own time and to their own priorities.

What do we mean by clinical intuition?

Greenhalgh (2002) describes intuition as a crucial and valid component of *expert decision-making*. Features of intuition are described as follows:

- it is a rapid, unconscious process
- it is context-sensitive
- it comes with practice

- it involves selective attention to small details
- it cannot be reduced to cause-and-effect logic (for example, B happened because of A)
- it addresses, integrates and makes sense of multiple and complex pieces of data.

The *novice* practitioner is characterized as someone who:

- adheres rigidly to taught rules or plans
- possesses little situational perception
- has no discretionary judgement.

The *competent* practitioner:

- is able to cope with 'crowdedness' and pressure
- sees actions partly in terms of long-term goals or a wider conceptual framework
- follows standardized and routinized procedures.

The *expert* practitioner:

- no longer relies explicitly on rules, guidelines and maxims
- has an intuitive grasp of situations based on deep, tacit understanding
- uses analytic (deductive) approaches only in novel situations or when problems occur.

This means that an expert practitioner intuitively tends to demonstrate a high level of listening skills and a relaxed ability to explore relevant issues. They need to be sensitive to the verbal and non-verbal cues from all family members. They also need to have the confidence to explain carefully why it is relevant to explore so many issues. Although confidence will come from having listened to the experiences of many bereaved families, practitioners will need to develop a set of skills informed by a theoretical framework (Bentovim and Bingley Miller 2001).

The assessment requires the ability to stay with a difficult subject for some time and not be diverted into talking about something more comfortable. If the family appears uncomfortable with a certain line of questioning then the practitioner needs to draw on his or her skills to gently reframe their questions. It is crucial that the parent or child does not feel 'judged' and feels sufficiently secure at least to reflect on the issues being raised.

A training manual supported by the Department of Health – *The Family Assessment: Assessment of Family Competence, Strengths and Difficulties* – is an excellent resource for practitioners seeking further guidance on how to complete a systemic assessment (Bentovim and Bingley Miller 2001).

Method of assessment

The assessment needs to consider the child within his or her *family system*. Secondly, it aims to consider the impact of the death on the wider *community system* – for example, school, friends, religious institution, sports clubs, and so on – and thirdly it assesses the *situational factors* arising from the death itself: for example, if the death was by suicide. The determinants of grief (see page 30) also provide a clear framework to understand the unique grief response of individuals within the family system. Much of the information-gathering begins through drawing up a genogram.

Genograms have several functions in a bereavement assessment:

- On a purely practical level genograms provide a written account of *who is who* in the family. It improves communication and trust significantly when family members can be referred to using their family names and other details.

- Genograms help to identify *previous losses* – for example, deaths, divorce, chronic illness, disability and unemployment – and to gauge their severity based on the perceptions of family members.

- Genograms also allow the practitioner to identify how the family has *coped with such previous losses*. They can explore which coping strategies were positive and helpful, and identify potential trends that proved unhelpful. For example, a parent might say: 'When I lost my job I suppose I turned to drinking quite heavily' and, in response, questions such as: 'Have you found yourself drinking more since Marion's death?' may be legitimately explored.

- Finally, the genogram can be used to determine the impact of the death on the *current family system*. In particular, are there any *key transitions* for this family, such as moving schools, marital separations, emigrations, weddings, retirements, serious illness in another family member, conflict relationships, dependency issues or other current or imminent issues? It is a reasonable hypothesis to assume that a family coping with the death of a parent or sibling will find such transitions an additional burden.

As well as the genogram itself, children's self-esteem, knowledge of issues relating to death and bereavement, capacity or willingness to remember, and their relationships with peers, teachers and others need to be explored.

Throughout the general assessment process the practitioner needs to be mindful of the factors which may have promoted *resilience* throughout childhood (Newman 2002, 2003) (see Table 3.2).

Table 3.2

Assessing resilience in childhood

- Strong social support networks
- The presence of at least one unconditionally supportive parent or parent substitute
- Positive school experiences
- A sense of mastery and a belief that one's own efforts can make a difference
- Participation in events outside school and the home
- The capacity to reframe adversities so that the beneficial effects are recognized
- The ability – or the opportunity – to make a difference by helping others or through part-time work (for teenagers).
- Not to be excessively sheltered from challenging situations which provide opportunities to develop coping skills.

(Newman 2003)

Table 3.3

The significant seven characteristics of bereaved children	Five personality traits or predispositions of resilient children
External locus of control	Internal locus of control
Lower self-esteem	Healthy self-esteem
Higher levels of anxiety/fearfulness	Easy-going temperament
Higher evidence of depression	Affectionate
More accidents and health problems	Good reasoning skills
Pessimism about the future	
Under performing	

Shuurman (2003) developed a comparison of bereaved children and resilient children (see Table 3.3).

Shuurman believes: 'the key at-risk factor bereaved children demonstrate in greater proportion than their nonbereaved peers is an external locus of control. Resilient children have a strong belief that they can control their fates by their own actions; bereaved children show a higher evidence of externalizing control, believing that their fate is in someone else's hands. No wonder they display higher levels of anxiety, depression, pessimism, health problems, underperformance, and lower self-esteem' (Shuurman 2003).

Before the assessment

Research consistently shows that it is not easy for parents to connect emotionally to their children's grief (Dyregrov 1991). However, the literature also concludes that parents often have the greatest influence on their child's adjustment (Silverman 2000). It is therefore absolutely crucial to fully engage the parent or carer, and for them to feel confident with the assessment process. It can be helpful to telephone a parent before a home visit to check if there are any issues they are concerned about discussing in front of the children. This can liberate a parent reluctant to access services because they feel paralyzed by a 'secret', for example: 'I can't face telling the children that their brother killed himself... not yet anyway'. In time, we would usually hope to work towards a family understanding of the suicide – however, it is very important that the parent feels in control of the information-sharing process. It is not the role of a child bereavement service to 'take over' and enforce principles of open, honest discussion before the time feels right for the parent.

Allocating sufficient time

Family assessment can be a key intervention in itself and ideally should not feel rushed. It takes time to build rapport, in order to share emotional information and get a realistic sense of how the family relates. Time is also needed to tell the family about the range of services on offer. It is usually helpful to see each member of the family individually as well as assessing how the family functions together. At Winston's Wish up to half a day is usually allocated for a full assessment. This includes travelling time and time to write up the notes.

The importance of engaging the whole family

Parents may need to keep their children home from school so that the whole family gets the most out of the assessment. As the school will need an explanation for absence this can provide an opportunity to reinforce the school's awareness that a child in its care is coping with a significant bereavement.

In family discussions when the children are present, practitioners need to take care to use words that children can understand so that they do not feel excluded.

The home setting

Assessments which take place in a family's home will need to follow policy guidelines addressing the health and safety issues involved in home visiting. When it is time for the children to be interviewed, the practitioners ask them where they would like to talk. This is often their bedroom, or a separate room downstairs. Parental consent must be given for any room used. Doors should be left open and child protection guidelines followed.

Absent family members

Practitioners also need to plan how they will respond if key family members are missing. There is a balance between affirming and working with those who attend while explaining how difficult it is to get to know the family as a whole without the presence and perspective of key members. Asking a family's views about how the absent member(s) might respond to a further invitation to attend can be a good way of exploring family realities (Bentovim and Bingley Miller 2001).

Family members who are reluctant to join in

Sometimes a parent might say: 'Simon is home, but he is in his room and doesn't want to come down'. In such situations it can be useful to ask who in the family would be best at persuading the child to come in, and perhaps sending them to see the child with a message from you. The approach could be something like this: 'Am I right in thinking Simon is upstairs and not sure about joining us? Could someone in the family go and say from me that it would be great if he could join us, even for a short while? Who would be best to do that?'

Framework for a home assessment

Although each home assessment is tailored to meet each individual family's needs, the visit is likely to take place flexibly within the following framework.

Understanding the reason for the visit

With all the family together, the practitioners will need to check that the child(ren) know about the reason for the visit.

Rationale for assessment

It is necessary to ensure that the child(ren) understand that the visit is not because they have been naughty or are 'sick' but that it is quite natural and usual to help when an important person in someone's life has died.

Referrer

If the parent was not the referrer then it may be appropriate to talk about the person who made contact, and their connections with the family.

Explaining the assessment format

Starting on time, and continuing to keep to the agreed time boundaries, is one indication to the family that you will work professionally and respectfully with them. It tells the family that they can rely on you to keep the agreements you make with them. A balance is needed between formality and informality which recognizes that the practitioner and the family have some important work to do together.

In explaining the format for the visit the practitioner could suggest for a family with a mother and two children (called John and Vicky): 'What we would like to do now is suggest that perhaps I have a chance to talk with mum on her own. John, perhaps you could meet with my colleague Jim? That means that Vicky can have a break for half an hour until John and Jim have finished. Does that sound OK? When we've finished we will all catch up together as a family and we can talk about the ways we may be able to help'.

Establishing rapport

When making an assessment of the emotional, cognitive, and behavioural issues arising from the death, an experienced practitioner will confidently and carefully explain *why* it is necessary to explore these avenues. The parent or child needs to feel *in control* of what information they choose to share. Questioning should be objective and non-judgemental. For example, asking about 'your partner' rather than 'your husband' might make it easier to explain that a couple were not married or that their partner was the same sex. Similarly, a practitioner gently exploring the meaning a wife is giving to her husband's fatal drink-driving road traffic accident might say: 'If I am hearing you correctly–it seems that most people were very surprised that John's post-mortem suggested he had been drinking quite heavily. Did it come as a surprise to you?'

Utilizing a family tree to gather information

As mentioned previously, a useful way to begin the assessment is to construct a family tree or *genogram* (Dobson 1989). The symbols used when constructing a family tree are shown in Fig. 3.1. If the children appear reluctant to leave their parent then it

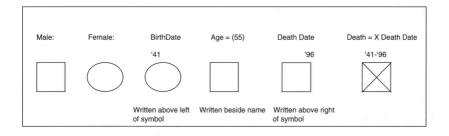

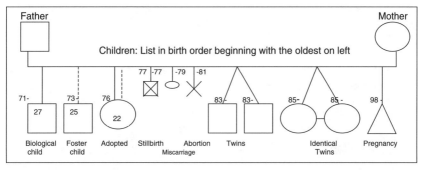

Fig. 3.1 Example of symbols of use when constructing a family tree.

can be informative to do the family tree with the children present. Children often enjoy doing this, and it can give the practitioner valuable insights into how the family functions. For example, it becomes clear how much the children know about their family, how the parent(s) and children communicate with each other, and the level of respect each shows for the other in the way they give and share information. Some parents speak for their children while others encourage them to work out the family relationships and everyone's ages for themselves, only helping out when necessary.

It is usually helpful to have different colours or symbols for male and female, for people who are alive and those who have died and so on. It is also useful to put dates on for deaths and separations, including divorces. The practitioner may want to invite the family to show, again through symbols or colours, who is especially close or has particularly distant or ambivalent relationships – see Fig. 3.2. The discussion can focus on a range of aspects using these techniques. Finding out what influence the family perceives other members from past generations have had on them can provide useful and interesting information. Asking who takes after whom can help to identify ways in which the family members are bringing forward their understanding of the past. Asking children how much they know about past generations or their extended family can give a sense of how much the immediate family identifies and feels part of the rest of the family, past and present. This may also present an insight into how motivated

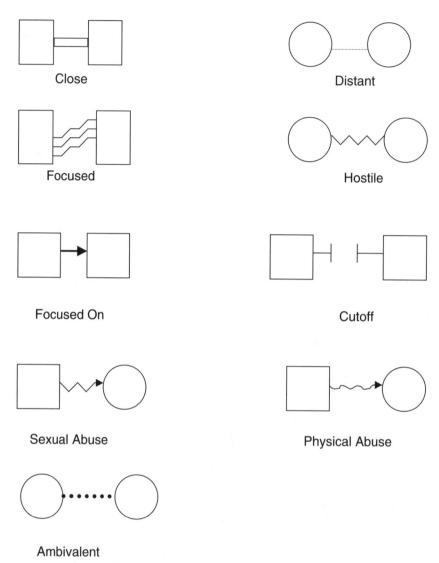

Fig. 3.2 Symbols denoting type of relationship.

parents are at helping to preserve memories. 'Mum says that I am just like grandad, always grumpy and picky with my food.'

However, it is likely that the parent will, at times, decide to protect the children from certain information. If the genogram is completed with the children present, the practitioner will need to check out later if there was anything that the parent had chosen not to mention in front of the children. A parent might then say, for example: 'I didn't like to mention this in front of Becky, but my husband was actually married before and so Becky has a half sister' or 'The children don't know but I had just petitioned for divorce.

He had been unfaithful but now he's died I don't want it to affect the kids' memory of their dad'.

In constructing a genogram the practitioner will also try to establish family members' own perspective of themselves and to see how far they recognize their strengths and difficulties. This can provide a useful insight into the resilience demonstrated by the family as a whole. A great deal can be gleaned by the way family members talk about their perception of their strengths and difficulties. It also gives an indication of the degree to which the relationships in the family are supportive and appreciative, or otherwise, and how the family attributes strengths and difficulties. 'Even though dad has died we are still a family.'

The following case study provides an overview of the process outlined in constructing a genogram. In particular, it is intended to show careful cross-referencing, establishing the 'meaning' which each family member gives to the 'facts' as they emerge.

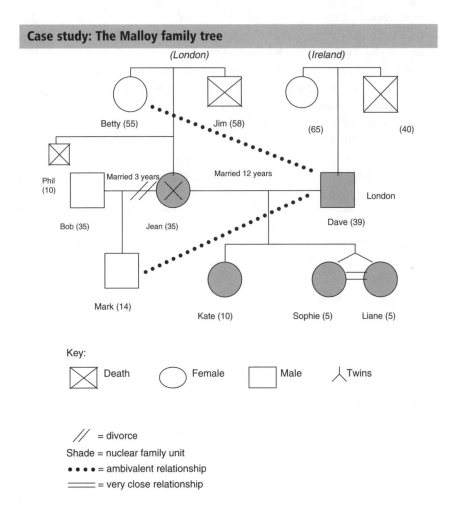

Case study: The Malloy family tree

By constructing a genogram, the practitioner would quickly identify a number of key facts and issues, a few of which are listed below. Taken in isolation these facts tell us very little: the richness comes when the *meaning and relevance of these issues to various family members* have been discussed in order to complete the picture of interwoven threads.

The following information was obtained when drawing the genogram with the children's father (Dave):

- Dave and Jean had been married for 12 years and they had three daughters. Jean had been married before: the marriage lasted three years and she had a son (Mark) from the marriage who is now 14.
- Jean died in a road traffic accident. She was not driving; the driver survived. Jean was not wearing a seatbelt. She was 35 years old.
- Kate was a passenger and witnessed her mother's death. She is showing symptoms of post-traumatic stress.
- Kate is in her last year at primary school. She will change to a secondary school in September.
- Dave is currently thinking that this might be a good time to make a fresh start by moving closer to his mother who lives in Ireland.
- Dave's father died suddenly aged 40. Dave was 8 at the time, and he will be 40 next year.
- Mark, a step-brother, has a volatile relationship with his step-dad (Dave) which worsened significantly when his mother died.
- After Jean's death Mark decided to move back to live with his father. He is still local and hasn't changed school.
- Sophie and Liane are together in the reception year at school. Jean had decided with the school that the twins would go into separate classes after completion of their reception year.
- Dave has a complicated relationship with Jean's mother, who has expressed her belief that he is 'too busy' with his job to care properly for the children. She helps with household chores and insists that all Jean's things remain in place.
- Betty is devastated by her daughter's death but seems hard to reach and needs to blame others.
- Betty is in close contact with Mark.
- Betty's husband (Jean's father) died last year. The cause of death was confirmed as suicide, from carbon monoxide poisoning in a car. Jim had struggled with depression since his son's death from leukaemia 20 years earlier. He died on his son's birthday.
- The children were told that their grandfather had had an accident in the car. Dave said he felt uncomfortable with this explanation as it was misleading.
- Bob (Jean's first husband) enjoyed a good relationship with both Jean and Dave. 'They married young, had Mark, but split up when he was a baby.' Bob lives close by and tries to build bridges between Mark and Dave.

These are just *some* of the many issues which emerged, helping the practitioner to build a picture of the impact of Jean's death, at this particular time, for this particular family, living in this particular community.

The smaller picture

Understanding different viewpoints – illustrated by taking one specific issue arising from this assessment

The practitioner's role is to establish *facts* and then try to understand their *meaning* for different family members. *It is not just the actual facts themselves which determine risk – it is the meaning that different family members give to them.* Using an example from this genogram we could reflect on the meaning different people might have for the seemingly inconsequential plan to separate the twins when they return for their second year at school. While this had been agreed with Jean, as part of the school's policy, the plan took on a different meaning for different people after her death.

Dave's view

Since Jean's death Dave is desperate to make sure that the family feels safe and secure. He says Jean was really good at this and he sometimes feels he doesn't know where to start. He is anxious that nothing unnecessary should upset the balance of family life. Dave remembers a long period of refusing to go to school when his father died. His mother was happy for him to stay at home and responded protectively to even fairly minor physical symptoms. Dave is worried that the girls are starting to do the same, and he knows this will be difficult with his work. 'I just want to do my best for the girls. At times I feel like running away because it's all too much. The twins being put into separate classes is the final straw!' Dave says that he feels furious with the school and strongly believes that regular stomach aches experienced by the twins are connected to their worries about being separated from him and each other.

Sophie's view

Sophie seems to have become more dependent on Liane; she is unusually aggressive. Sophie says she is scared that boys at school will make jokes about the fact that her mum has died. 'I want to be with my sister, always.'

Liane's view

The quieter twin, she frequently wets herself at school and is rarely vocal, allowing her sister to speak on her behalf. Liane whispered to the practitioner: 'I wish my dad could give up work so I can stay at home, or perhaps mum can come back from heaven'.

The school's view

With Dave's permission, the school was telephoned after the home assessment. The head teacher explained that he has not yet personally spoken to Dave about the twins. 'Dave has got so much on his plate that I don't want to burden him further at the moment. I'd be happy to talk about next year when he is ready.' The girls' class teacher believes that Liane would benefit from greater independence from Sophie, but is reluctant to say this to Dave as she senses his vulnerability and quick temper. So, it would appear that a breakdown in communication has meant that Dave now perceives the school as being cold and inflexible, and gives him further evidence for his belief that he is isolated and vulnerable.

So, it is only after the practitioner has gleaned an understanding from various perspectives that they can then try to generate a hypothesis about what is going on and how a seemingly small issue, such as the twins' school attendance, needs to be moved forward or resolved in a positive way while the family is in crisis.

The bigger picture

Assessing risk and resilience

The overall assessment revealed a variety of issues which informed the practitioners how past family history affects and how different family members are coping with Jean's death. In addition, it identified the impact of her death having occurred at this particular time: for example, Kate will soon be changing to secondary school, Dave is considering moving to Ireland, the twins had just started school and it is only a year since the maternal grandfather died by suicide. Family members hold differing views on the factors which led to both the grandfather's and Jean's deaths.

The assessment process aims to unravel how different family members reacted to previous losses and, again, to relate this to the current situation. For example, while Dave was understanding about Betty's devastation following the deaths of her children and husband, he felt frustrated by her emotional outbursts and angry that she couldn't offer more practical help with child care. He also felt that Betty intensified the difficulties he had in relating to Mark.

While the assessment is about collecting information, it can also become an intervention in itself especially if the practitioner uses techniques (such as circular questioning) to loosen family assumptions. For example, questions such as 'Who do you think is most upset about mum's death? If I asked dad if he was thinking of moving to Ireland what do you think he would say? If granny Betty could have three wishes what do you think they would be? If you could have three wishes what would you ask for? If I had met your family before mum died, what would an average week have been like?' could be asked.

At the end of 2–3 hours the assessment was completed. The family reported feeling both exhausted but relieved to have spoken so openly and honestly.

Sharing information with the rest of the family

The family regroups once all the individual interviews have taken place. It is important for everyone to check out what information they are willing to have shared when the family unit 'regroups'. Sometimes the practitioners will need to reframe ideas for the children: this may enable the children to share something in a way that they believe will be more acceptable to their parent. For example, the practitioner might say: 'You know you said that your mum is always shouting and angry since your dad died … when we meet back up with mum would it be OK to say something like: "The children have noticed that you sometimes seem to be more irritable and tired since their dad died, and they were wondering if they could help in any way?"'

Closing the assessment and leaving the family with a task

If appropriate, families are introduced to the possibility of choosing or developing their own memory box. The rationale is explained, and children and parents are invited to share ideas on how they might build up the contents of their own individual box. This exercise provides a stimulating closing activity for the assessment and, in addition, leaves a tangible attachment and reminder of the purpose of meeting with the family.

Planning appropriate interventions

Before leaving, the practitioner will give a broad outline of what they think might be the best way forward. In terms of the programme available at Winston's Wish this could be a combination of some of the following (see Fig. 3.3):

(a) family invited to attend a residential weekend

(b) discussion with a child's teacher or any other significant agency

(c) individual work with the parent

(d) individual work with a child

(e) invitation for the family to attend a group: our current group programmes particularly focus on families affected by suicide or a group for families with pre-school aged children

(f) referral to another agency

(g) no further contact.

This chapter has explored the ways in which a detailed assessment can guide the most appropriate intervention for each family. Assessment of family functioning, and of the wider context in which a child exists, is one of the hardest yet most important skills a practitioner has to develop. The well-being of bereaved children depends on our being able to identify those strengths within a family on which we can build, and to define those difficulties we are aiming to help alleviate. There are many effective ways to bring up children, so any approach must be non-judgemental and flexible to respect that variety.

Three key points are raised:

◆ A comprehensive assessment involves the bereaved child, their parent(s) and the community in which the child lives.

◆ The assessment is used to establish the needs of this particular family and plan appropriate interventions.

◆ Practitioners will need a range of skills which enable them to hold assessment criteria in their head while being intuitively responsive to subtle signals from the child and/or parent. The assessment can be viewed as an intricate dance, where the practitioner may well know the 'steps' but has the confidence to allow the 'rhythm' to be determined by the family.

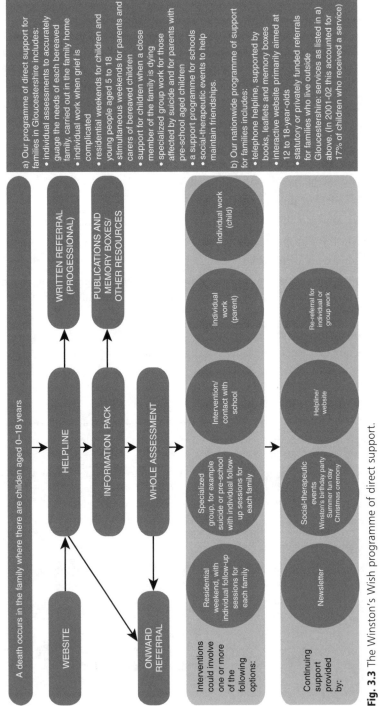

Fig. 3.3 The Winston's Wish programme of direct support.

References

Bentovim A, Bingley Miller L (2001). *The family assessment: assessment of family competence, strengths and difficulties.* Brighton: Pavilion Publishing.

Dobson S (1989). Genograms and Ecomaps. *Nursing Times, Nursing Mirror* December 26; **85**(51):54.

Dyregrov A (1991). *Grief in children: A handbook for adults.* London: Jessica Kingsley.

Glaser D, Furniss T, Bingley L (1984). Focal Family Therapy: The Assessment Stage. *Journal of Family Therapy* 4:132–77.

Greenhalgh T (2002). Uneasy bedfellows? Reconciling intuition and evidence-based practice. *Young Minds Magazine* **59**:23–7.

Newman T (2002). *Promoting resilience: a review of effective strategies for child care services.* University of Exeter: Centre for Evidence Based Social Sciences: www.exeter.ac.uk/cebss

Newman T (2003). Protection racket. *Zero2Nineteen* (January issue):8.

Parkes CM, Weiss RS (1983). *Recovery from bereavement.* New York: Basic Books, pp. 31–4.

Schuurman D (2003). *Never the same – coming to terms with the death of a parent.* New York: St Martin's Press, pp. 130–1.

Shapiro ER (1994). Grief as a family process: A developmental approach to clinical practice. New York: Guilford Press.

Silverman PR (2000). *Never too young to know: death in children's lives.* New York: Oxford University Press.

Chapter 4

The family perspective in bereavement

Peta Hemmings

Introduction

In this chapter, the nature of a therapeutic social work service for families living with serious illness and bereavement has been outlined. Following on from this, two case studies are presented, one is a brief intervention with a family and the second is an intervention with a child and his brother several years after their mother's death.

Responding to vulnerable families

For many families the death of a family member is the first collective crisis. The extent of the impact and the intensity of the experience may, for the first time, lead them to seek professional help. The combination of these two factors have a tendency to make the parents, who are usually the active agents at this stage, feel less rather than more competent and less in control of the family's situation. The process of recognizing the need for additional resources and the act of seeking them can further undermine an already shaky foundation. It is therefore vitally important that the manner in which the service is described, presented and delivered, from the initial stages onwards, is perceived by the parent as a positive experience.

One of the key elements in this process lies in an explicit recognition of the parent's personal strengths, the family's inherent resourcefulness and their achievements to date. These are the working tools of all interventions, without which few therapeutic techniques will have effect.

Process as product

It is a given that, no matter how we examine and audit our work, no therapeutic service is flawless. Secondly, we need to acknowledge that no service can meet all the needs of all families. This is not a 'get out' clause but a reasonable and necessary starting point. I emphasize this because the effectiveness of a therapeutic service is based on having a clear understanding of what is possible in the context of a reliable, organized system of responses to enquiries and referrals.

The baseline is a considered referral criterion based on a clear understanding of the remit of the agency matched with recognition of the skills within the team. For example, my practice base, the Bereavement and Serious Illness Team within Barnardo's Orchard Project, is primarily a social work service working with families, living in the north-east region of England, who have been affected by the death of a family member or another significant relationship. We accept referrals from a wide range of agencies within the physical and mental health services, educational communities, social service departments, and directly from families themselves. The team conducts an initial assessment of the family's needs and, where appropriate, usually offers a short-term or brief therapeutic intervention. However, the fact that a referral fulfils these criteria does not mean that our team would automatically undertake all the work identified by the initial assessment.

Partly because our resources are limited and partly because we are a social work service, we would not accept sole responsibility for therapeutic work with families referred where it was clear that, for example, there were additional mental health difficulties, longstanding parenting issues or other areas of work outwith our skills or resources. Our focus is primarily on issues related to or arising from the serious illness or bereavement. Although it is not easy to say that this or that feature of an individual's behaviour or emotional state is attributable to one or other identifiable cause, it is reasonable to assume that if a family had a history of parenting problems pre-dating the bereavement, which continued to be a feature after the death, then this behaviour is not specifically loss-related and, consequently, not something that would necessarily warrant our involvement except in relation to the bereavement-related work in hand. Having identified the issue, however, it may be desirable for another service, for whom it is their specific remit, to become or remain involved.

It is essential to be clear about what can and cannot be offered and to identify service limitations. It is a practice strength and part of establishing an open and honest contract with the family. Having a distinct professional identity is the starting point for enhanced effectiveness. When the role of an agency is clear, it is more likely that neither the family nor the worker has unrealistic expectations of themselves or the service. This approach also makes it easier to identify the appropriateness of engaging partner agencies to pick up the other aspects of the work or carry on supporting the family after involvement with the Orchard Project has closed.

An immediate response

A seminal element in the process of intervention is the parent's and child's experiences of their first contact with the service. The act of telephoning and speaking to a stranger about emotionally painful and personal matters can make a parent feel even more vulnerable. Recognizing the need and plucking up the courage to ask for help is sometimes a difficult process in itself. Making that move to contact an agency, leaving a message and not hearing from anyone for several days may have all sorts of meaning for the parent, ranging from regret at exposing themselves in this way to anger that nobody is recognizing and responding to their need for support.

In recognition of this, Orchard Project offers a rapid response to any initial contact, but with particular attention to calls which are from parents or non-professionals. Team members set aside, on a rota basis, several blocks of time during the course of a working week, to respond to incoming calls and give time to listen to parents' concerns about their children and explore ways in which they think they can be best supported to help their children. Information about how the parent identifies the difficulties and is managing the situation is collected along with information about existing supportive resources, including extended family, friends, schools, and other agencies. In this way the parent is encouraged to think through what resources are currently available and their ideas about how effective or otherwise strategies they have already tried have been. The initial assessment is conducted from a position of reviewing the resourcefulness and emphasizing the achievements of parents rather than concentrating on the problem to the exclusion of all else.

The orientation of a strengths-based rather than a problem-based perspective establishes the culture of the service from the first conversation onwards. The amount of crises that have been effectively managed often comes as something of a surprise to a parent, boosting a flagging sense of competence and confidence. Even in the bleakest landscape of family life there are some green shoots if we look hard enough. These are the family's seminal resources around which we can start to encourage further growth and development.

This solution focused view of family work is rapidly gaining ground in mental health and social work services. In their review of Child and Adolescent Mental Health services in South Australia, Nichols and Schwartz (1995) observe that '... the orientation towards solutions ... is an attempt to create an atmosphere in which people's strengths can move out of the shadows and into the foreground.'

The approach of responding quickly, listening attentively and encouraging the parent to think about all that they have managed till date helps create a positive experience. From the very start the parent is defined as an active agent in developing additional resources for the family based on his or her assessment of the family's need. At this point the parent is the expert in relation to their children's needs and a partner in whatever work may follow. Allison *et al.* (2003) state that, 'There is an increasing body of work in the psychotherapy literature on the importance of 'common factors' that account for variance in therapeutic outcome. ... The concept of personal and family strengths as a critical focus is repeated consistently throughout ....'

Assessment process

If the initial referral information indicates that there are difficulties which the parent is either unable to manage at that time or which are too complex or too sensitive to discuss indirectly, then a home visit is arranged and a fuller assessment of the family's circumstances follows.

Unless there are confidential issues to be discussed, it is usual for the parent to be encouraged to ask the children if they would like to be present. Children often have a very different perspective on what is the problem and it is not uncommon for the presence of a professional outsider to facilitate a freer sharing of views, which can help move things on for the family. It is important that the assessment process is conducted in ways which make it part of the overall therapeutic experience, not merely an information gathering exercise. In order to make it more relevant and inclusive of children I use a range of drawing or play-based activities alongside the conversational element.

I referred earlier to some of the resources and areas of family functioning which are assessed as part of the initial contact. A fuller assessment would explore in more detail individual experiences of events leading up to and including the death and how they were managed. If one child within the sibling group was the focus of the parent's concern, the reasons why this is so would be explored alongside the meaning it has for the parent. This can be a very fruitful and illuminating area because it may reveal the discreet or unconscious significance to the parent of the child's behaviour (Reder and Duncan 1995). It is not unusual for family myths or qualities attributed or projected onto the child to become apparent, all of which have bearing upon which type of intervention would be most appropriate. There are several markers to be drawn from an assessment which inform the decision about which intervention is the method of choice but it is essentially a sliding scale or continuum of professional judgement. At one end of the continuum, it would be highly inappropriate to offer individual work with a child who is seen as 'the problem'. To do so would endorse the child's role as the family's scapegoat and place an impossible burden on him to 'recover' through therapy and so 'heal' the family. Similarly it would not be appropriate to offer family work where it was clear that the parent's personal issues were the main focus. That is not to say that one method could not follow the other, consequently it is often the case that the outcome of the assessment is a recommendation that a package of services is offered, some of which may come from Orchard Project and some from other agencies.

Balancing family life

Communication is one of the commonest difficulties bereaved families experience. When someone dies after a long, degenerative illness so much has happened to the family on the way that parents and children are left physically and emotionally exhausted. For the parents it has often been a struggle managing childcare arrangements, organizing the household, attending to domestic tasks, getting to work, and keeping up to date with their children's activities and progress at school. The idea of having space in the daily timetable to enjoy being with the children may be a luxury they can little afford. The notion of having a period of calm, with no rushing to and from the hospital or up and down stairs with trays of food to a sick partner or child, may be a distant memory. As Bluebond-Langner (1996) observes: 'Chronic illness is woven into the fabric that is the life of the ill and their families.'

It is understandable that parents, aware of this imbalance in their family's life, are torn between their need to be with and caring for the ill person and their wish to have time for their children and other family members.

For children, the repeated experience of mini-crises erodes their sense of security in the world. Children are obliged to adapt, often without warning, to changes of plan. For example, coming out of school to find it is grandmother at the gates or a friend's mother who has come to collect them, is at least disconcerting if not worrying for children. Even though the adult may be well known to the child, the experience of another change of plan eats away at his sense of how reliable and predictable the world is. Many children quickly become anxious about what can happen at home when they are not there. It is this undercurrent of worry that washes over them from time to time and begins to pervade their world.

It is clear that, '... stressors rarely occur singly and, instead, may be seen as forming chains of primary and secondary stressors ...' (Gore and Eckenrode 1996). The protracted experience of sequential crises creates a sense of uncertainty about the world and profoundly undermines the family's collective sense of security. The societal context also has some bearing upon this process. Parents are often aware, whether explicitly or subconsciously, that their experience is not the norm. Other families are perceived as living in an increasingly different world of comparative order and good health. This perceived disparity may inhibit parents from sharing their worries with neighbours or other parents as they wait together at the school gates.

> Beginning at the macro level of the experience, one must never lose sight of the fact that well siblings and their families live in a society where chronic illness and disability are stigmatised, and normalcy, control and order are valued.
>
> Bluebond-Langner (p. 266)

The societal context becomes an increasingly important factor in the effect of the crises and one which adds to the final toll. It is not surprising that at the end, when the death has occurred and the flurry of activity around the funeral is over and the family starts to reform in its new shape and pull together new routines, there is a time of reckoning.

The process of re-creating a family life is not easy. A multitude of features affect how the family re-groups and establishes a new order, many of which are not in harmony or synchrony with one another. For example, variations in the parents' individual mourning styles may create distance rather than closeness in their relationship. Any ripples of unease between them are inevitably felt within the household. The manner in which children respond to loss is influenced by a range of factors including gender, personal style, and levels of developmental maturity (Dyregrov 1995). Children's episodic mourning pattern is significantly different to adults' style of mourning, which more closely represents a reactive depression. The difference in patterns of mourning between children and their parents is an additional factor which can create another strand of tension within the family. In addition, the surviving children suddenly find that for the first time in a long while they are the focus of their parents' attention. This may be a very mixed experience, ranging from pleasure at having their company to unease at the intensity of the experience. Layer upon layer of factors have to be accommodated.

The accumulative effects on the family of the illness crises combined with the personal impact on individual family members mean that the permutations for families are infinite. We may receive a referral for a family bereaved as a result of degenerative illness but, because the route to that point can be so varied, each one is unique, however, underpinning many referrals will be one of the commonest problems families experience, that of communication.

Families develop various ways of managing the intense threats posed by crises. In the following example I will outline how one family responded to family life that increasingly revolved around illness until it became the sole focus and how the death of the child left a void in their lives which neither parent could manage for the surviving child. Managing the aftermath is often as troubling as managing the illness.

Case study: The Harvey Family and the Rock Pool World

Family history

The Harvey family lived in a small village near the coast. Sue and Jim's first child, Mark, was a healthy baby and, when he was two years old, the couple were delighted to find that Sue was pregnant again. Jade was born and Sue and Jim felt their family was complete.

Jade was a healthy baby until, at fourteen months, she suffered a series of *grand mal* seizures. During the next six months she became progressively unwell and there were repeated emergency hospital admissions. Many of these crises developed during the night and Mark would wake to find his mother and Jade were gone and his father was tired and anxious. Sue often stayed in hospital with Jade for several days. Mark visited them but soon became bored and wanted to go home.

During the last three months of her life Jade was cared for largely at home by Sue with the support of community nursing services. Mark helped by doing little tasks like getting tissues or bowls of water. His grandmother came almost daily and took him out to the park or the beach. One day she commented on how quiet he had become. He no longer wanted to go on the swings at the park and usually stayed close by her rather than running around on the beach.

Jade died shortly before her third birthday. Sue told Mark she had become an angel in heaven and he could see her as a bright star in the night sky. He did not go to the funeral, but went out with a friend and his mother to the park and to MacDonalds.

The Immediate Aftermath

One year later Sue and Jim were having difficulties. Mark was very challenging at home and Sue admitted to having lost her patience and smacked him a couple of times. Jim disapproved of smacking and they had argued about it in front of Mark.

Sue was worried about the way Mark played, often engrossed in play with small figures but he stopped if she came in the room and would not let her join in. If she read to him he would sit beside her but not on her lap, as he used to, nor would he let her put her arm a round him. If he fell or hurt himself while playing he would not let either of them comfort him. Mark resisted going to bed without one of them beside him until he fell asleep and often woke in the night distressed by his dreams.

Mark's teacher commented that he was aggressive towards children at playtime and had taken and hidden pencils and other personal items belonging to classmates. Although it was manageable, she felt they should know it was becoming a feature of his behaviour in school.

Sue and Jim also felt they were less close. Jim worked full time and often went hill walking at the weekends: he said it helped him sort out his thoughts. Sue felt lonely at home: she saw her mother daily but not her friends because most of them had children who were the same age as Jade would have been and it was too painful for her to be around them.

Sue declined the offer of anti-depressants from her GP. A friend suggested bereavement counselling for Mark and Sue contacted Orchard Project. The whole family were involved in the initial assessment which took place over two sessions.

Assessment

It was apparent from the information that emerged that Sue and Jim were struggling to remain close to one another. They felt they were drifting apart at a time when they both needed emotional support but of different sorts which neither was able to provide for the other. They were unable to talk about Jade's illness and avoided any reference to her death. They shared few activities and were often irritable with one another when together.

Mark was aware of the underlying tension between his parents and was anxious about what this might lead to. He indicated his concern obliquely by several references to his friend who lived with his mother and saw his father every other weekend. He also referred to his change of status; no longer being a brother and being the only child. He liked the fact that family and friends had given him lots of presents and treats after Jade died, but did not understand why. He was confused about why Jade died and worried about what could happen next.

The assessment indicated that the underlying issue to be addressed was the quality of emotional communication within the family. The recommendation of family work, rather than individual work for Mark, was accepted and a series of four sessions was arranged over the course of the next six weeks.

Creating a family metaphor

Play is children's working vocabulary: it is their natural way to communicate without words. The challenge when working with families where communication is the main difficulty is to find a shared vocabulary that creates bridges between the individuals – which is where the use of metaphor comes in.

The Harveys' habit of going to the beach together provided the shared experience upon which to build the imagery. It is important to find a symbolic world with which each person connects because this facilitates exploration of the feelings and helps elucidate the dynamics of family relationships. Having agreed that going to the beach and rooting around in rockpools was something they enjoyed, I set about creating a Rock Pool World (see Fig. 4.1).

Materials

I stapled two large sheets of sugar paper together, one a dull yellow, onto which I glued patches of sand, and the other blue, and drew a cross-section of a rockpool (see Fig. 4.1). In the bottom of the pool were some small rocks, sea anemones, and strands of weed, some of which were made out of tissue paper. I glued a little flap of self-coloured paper on the sandy bottom of the pool. I drew a couple of small ledges at the sides. On the rim were some larger, flat rocks. In the blue sky above were a couple of seagulls. I made some cut-out clouds of white and grey and a sun and moon, which I kept separately.

The features of the rockpool lent themselves well to the purpose of the work. Like the family in their world, the rockpool is a boundaried, fixed entity yet ever-changing. The tide comes in and out, refreshing the water, bringing food and new creatures to the pool. Although the tides are predictable, their effect upon the creatures and plants varies according to their strength and environmental factors, like the weather and events elsewhere. Sometimes flotsam is washed up nearby; sometimes predatory

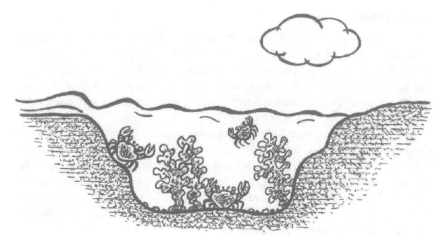

Fig. 4.1 The family rock pool.

creatures come by on the hunt. Seagulls wheel overhead and children come dipping with nets to see what they might find.

I made four paper crabs with little flaps on their backs. They were all the same size but different colours. I chose crabs because their physical qualities lent themselves to the issues which I anticipated could be central to the work. The crab is adapted to its environment, having a tough shell to protect it, agile legs to hold its food, and scuttle to safety when threatened, and it can survive in and out of water, blending in with the background when necessary. The addition of the flap on the back created an opportunity to think about how this well-adapted, defended creature is also vulnerable at times, carrying thoughts and feelings about the world which are not always visible.

In the following passages I will outline the course of work in the four sessions.

Session one: Creating a secure base and positive experiences

The family had asked for the sessions to be held at home and we initially spent some time setting the ground rules. This process not only establishes the need for boundaries to individual's behaviours but engages everyone in the experience of the work in hand. Each person was encouraged to contribute and I wrote down and, because Mark was pre-literate, illustrated each item, often with his help. The list was kept in a prominent place at each session, on the understanding that, with the group's agreement, anyone could add to the rules.

The Harveys' ground rules were that:

everyone listens when someone else is talking

nobody interrupts until the person talking has finished

everyone can say what they feel

nobody contradicts someone's feelings

nobody laughs at anyone's drawings

we stay in the room unless there is a need to leave e.g. lavatory break

we have a drinks break half way through the hour

telephones are turned off

we do not respond if someone knocks at the door

everything said and done in the session is private to the family and not to be repeated to anyone.

I added that I would record the sessions in accordance with the agency's recording standards and bring the record for the family to read or have read to them. I underlined that these records were confidential would be held securely in accordance with the limits of the Data Protection Act. I added the standard child protection rider to confidentiality, explaining carefully to Mark about the need to look after children and protect them from being hurt or frightened. We agreed that I would look after the artwork between sessions.

Establishing the ground rules is standard practice in family sessions. In large families it is important to ensure that each person has an opportunity to say something about how sessions will be conducted, no matter how small that detail may be. This approach enacts the principle that the means whereby an intervention is presented is as important as the experience itself. When we are looking at how to deliver therapeutic services, the process is the product.

A secondary function of setting ground rules is that it creates an opportunity for the family to have a shared conversation about safe issues, to listen to one another and to be together with a common purpose. The process models the culture of sessional work and sets the scene for subsequent sessions. For the practitioner it provides an opportunity to observe the family as a group: who sits where, who is on time, late or absent, what non-verbal communication passes between different members, what roles have been allocated or adopted by different people and so on. In the Harvey family it was interesting that, like me, Mark sat on the floor while his parents stayed in their armchairs. Later on, Jim moved onto the floor but Sue remained in her chair.

Having finished the ground rules. I presented the rock pool picture. We spent some time looking at it and talking about the beach and what they did there. Mark sensed there was more to it than this and was keen for us to move on, so I showed them the crabs and asked them to choose one. Mark chose a blue one and immediately discovered the flap on its back and excitedly showed it to his parents. Sue asked Jim to choose one for her. He chose a yellow one and a green one for himself, leaving the pink crab in the box.

I asked them to think of something they liked about themselves and write or draw it on a small square of paper and pop it under the flap on their crab. Mark set to, quickly writing and drawing with his arm round his paper. Jim thought briefly and wrote something down. Sue said she could not think of anything and asked Jim to help her out. Mark piped up that she was good at making cakes, drew a cake and gave it to her. Jim said she had a good sense of humour and, although Sue said she did not think so, she wrote it down reluctantly and put it under the flap.

I then asked them to write or draw something they liked about each other. They gave their compliments to each other in turn. Mark told his mother she made the best dinners and his father that he was brilliant in goal when they played football.

Jim said that Mark was a lovely boy and full of energy; he added the rider that he would like him to be less 'naughty' at home. I reminded Jim that this was about saying something positive and he withdrew the comment – but it had been heard. He said he liked the way Sue kept the house clean and organized. Sue complimented Mark for getting ready for school in the mornings and Jim for helping with the shopping.

By the time we had finished this exercise the hour was up. When they reviewed the session Jim observed that had been one of the few occasions they had been together for an hour without the television on and that he had enjoyed it. Sue agreed and was surprised how quickly the time had passed. Mark said he wanted another session tomorrow because he liked the crabs. We made another appointment for the following week.

Session two: The tide comes in and the family swims together

Mark welcomed me at the door and told me he had been drawing his crab and was looking forward to seeing it again and that he had made a sign for the front door, so his friends would know he was busy.

We spent the first few minutes reviewing everyone's thoughts and feelings about the first session, which seemed overall to have been a positive experience, allaying any fears Sue had about how it might have been. I asked them in turn what was better since we last met. Mark's grandmother been given him a toy car; Jim and Mark had visited the rock pools on the beach and flown Mark's kite. Sue had made a family dinner on Sunday and enjoyed eating together. Mark listened attentively to his parents talking about these positive family experiences.

During the course of this session I asked the family to think about what it would be like to be a crab in the rock pool when the tide was coming in. Mark was excited at the idea of the waves making eddies for him to ride on, like the ones at the leisure pool. Jim said the waves might bring some food for him to eat but they might also bring something that wanted to eat him. Mark suggested it might be a shark! His parents were amused by this idea. Sue said everything would shift about and it would be difficult to see through the swirling sand and seaweed. Mark suggested she used a snorkel and face mask.

I then asked them to think about what their crab needed in order to enjoy or manage that experience. Mark said he wanted to swim around in the water. He placed his crab on the edge of the rocks and dived in. Jim put his crab on the bottom of the pool, hiding it behind some of the weed. Sue placed hers on the ledge halfway down saying this was a good vantage point to spot danger. We spent a few minutes looking at the sculpt. Mark's crab swooped about in the swirling water whilst his parents' crabs huddled for safety under the seaweed or on patrol on the narrow ledge.

Sue said she needed to be on the ledge because she was worried about what bad thing could happen next. Her anxiety made her fearful and angry that she could not swim with Mark. Mark swam his crab down to the ledge and said she could join him. Sue's crab swam with him for a short while before returning to the ledge.

Jim said it made him happy seeing Sue and Mark swimming together and sad that they could not do it more often. I asked him where he would like to be in the rock pool. He moved his crab from behind the weed and onto the bottom of the rock pool. He said he wanted to swim with Sue and Mark but needed to look out because he knew there were predators about. Mark said that Jim could easily nip the shark's nose with his pincers to make it go away. He swam down to Jim's crab, linked pincers and they swam together. Jim said how much he liked swimming with Mark. Sue started to cry. Mark looked at her for a few moments, left his crab and climbed onto her lap. They cuddled each other. Jim stayed looking at the crabs and then moved towards them and stroked Sue's hand, saying it was all right. After a few minutes Jim suggested they all needed a drink and we agreed to have a break. Mark stayed on his Mother's lap while Jim and I made the drinks.

Sue said she had cried because she was heart broken that Jade would never know what it was like to swim with them and sad for Mark that she could not swim with him. I brought out the fourth crab and asked them all to draw or write something and give it to the Jade crab. Mark drew a heart, said he missed her and hoped she could swim in heaven. Jim drew a heart with lightning saying how much he loved her and how angry he felt that she had been taken from them. Sue drew a broken heart.

I asked them to think about where the Jade crab should go in the rock pool. Mark wanted her in the water with him but thought she should go in the sky. His parents agreed and he placed her on one of the clouds. He said he wanted her to be warm and asked if he could leave the room to get some cotton wool. He made a cosy cotton wool cloud bed for his sister. We spent a few minutes talking about how Jade would feel knowing she was so missed and loved by her family.

The session was drawing to a close and I asked the family to think about something they could all do together before our next session. Mark wanted to go swimming with his parents and this was agreed.

Session three: Coping and caring

During this session we focused on what it was like for the three crabs to be apart from Jade. Mark was concerned that she was not lonely or cold. His parents reassured him that she would have lots of friends and that both his grandfathers were there to look after her. Sue said it made her heart ache to think of never seeing her again. Mark said she would see her when she went to heaven and Sue agreed, but that was such a long time to wait. Jim felt angry with God for not letting her live when there were so many bad people in the world. We explored these themes, thinking about how they managed, carrying these thoughts and feelings around with them every day.

Mark felt angry that other boys had sisters and brothers. When he was at school he saw them playing together at playtime. He said he wanted to go to school with Jade, show her where to hang her coat and play with her like they did. His parents listened as we thought about how he would have done this and what it meant to him not to be a 'big brother' anymore. Sue said he would always be a 'big brother' and Jade would always be in their family even though she could not be with them. Sue moved from her chair onto the floor beside Mark and put her arm round him.

Sue's statement and action was a pivotal point in the work. The ways they had listened and responded to each other during the sessions and built on that with activities

between sessions indicated they had made a significant shift in their emotional awareness. I checked this out with the family and they agreed that things felt different. I suggested that we review these differences next week with a view to thinking about closing
our work.

Session four: Managing another ending

This session revolved around how the crabs saw the future in their rock pool and what
they needed to manage adverse experiences.

They talked about how to spend time together. Mark wanted his mother to watch
him and his father play football in the garden and for them to go swimming together
again. Sue understood that Jim needed to go off by himself sometimes, which was all
right so long as they had time together too. Jim had enjoyed going swimming with
them both and wanted more times like that but needed time alone too.

In closing we reviewed how much we had done together and what memories they
would take from the experience. Mark wanted to keep his crab and the Jade crab so
they could play together. Jim appreciated having the time to be together in this way
and had heard lots of things about how Sue and Mark were feeling for the first time.
Sue realized how far she had drifted from her family and that she wanted to be closer
to them but it was hard sometimes because she felt so sad.

They planned another family activity for the coming weekend and we set a date, six
weeks later, when I would do a follow-up visit.

At this visit things had moved on again. Mark was sleeping well, he was less challenging at home and more settled at school. He said he felt happy and liked playing
with his friends. Sue and Jim said they were able to talk more freely about their feelings and the family were planning a holiday later that summer.

Summary

The aim of the intervention was not to make everything better but to facilitate a shift in
how family members perceived and responded to one another. The ways in which the
Harveys engaged with and continued the work between and after the sessions ended
were markers of their commitment to the process. The benefits were evident in the way
they were able to explore their experiences, recognize how Jade's illness and death had
affected them differently and express themselves through the medium of shared activity.

Focused activities

I have written elsewhere about specific activities and techniques relating to establishing the secure base within therapeutic work (Hemmings 1998b); the analysis and
management of anger (Hemmings 1999); exploring and developing a supportive emotional environment (Hemmings 1998a); retracing children's understanding of events
surrounding degenerative illness (Hemmings 2001a); assessing the child's perspective
on family relationships and dynamics (Hemmings 2001b); helping children develop
insight into the sources and effects of their emotions (Hemmings 1995). These exercises only have value when embedded in a secure and trusting relationship, whether
that is with the parent-carer or worker (Bell 2002).

Developing a therapeutic relationship with a worker is not a short process (Axline 1989; Wilson *et al.* 1992): the worker requires knowledge of the child's personal and family history, any previous experiences of such work and current status. The assessment process in relation to the need for intervention is discussed in more detail elsewhere in this volume. It is important to develop a sensitive awareness of the child's personal style within the work and let the child or young person set the pace. This is especially true for children who have endured chronic or acute stress or who have had traumatic experiences, whether that be exposure to domestic violence (Fantuzzo 1991; Edelson 1999; Humphreys and Mullender 2002); emotional, physical or sexual abuse (Miller 1992; Cattanach 1993; Glaser 1995), bereavement through suicide (Wertheimer 1991) or murder (Hendriks 1995). In order to survive, children develop a range of coping strategies. Some of these are adaptive in the short term, in that they sustain the child through stressful episodes or periods; however, it is often the case that what is effective in the short-term becomes maladaptive in the longer term (Radke-Yarrow 1992; Langrock 2002). A sensitive awareness of the value to the child of the elaborate defensive strategies he may have created (Wilson 1992; Dyregrov 1995; Yule 2000) is central to the effectiveness of any therapeutic intervention. To extend Bowlby's analogy (1988), we should not open the door of the child's fortress before he feels safe enough to look at the emotional jungle.

Many of the children referred to the Orchard Project have experienced troubled early years and traumatic bereavements. Some have witnessed the death of one or more members of their family in a traffic incident: some are survivors of the same event and survival often has a particular resonance of guilt and chance. Some have found the body of the parent who has committed suicide in the family home. Some have been present when one parent murdered the other. All have intensely distressing images etched into their memories; many have found ways of defending themselves from the power of these memories but at a cost. Therapy does not make memories go away but the experience can start the process whereby the effects become more manageable. Children who have had this sort of bereavement usually require longer-term intervention because of the complexity of their defences.

Mourning and resolution of loss has a developmental component. A very young child can only manage so much and may need to return to the work at different developmental stages in order to re-think his experience and locate it in his contemporary world. In my second case study I will outline how a boy returned to his bereavement issues six years after the death of his mother.

Case study: Paul's developmental mourning timetable

Family background

Paul's (aged 10) mother, Jill, died six months after the birth of his brother, David. Jill's cancer had been masked and accelerated by the pregnancy. Paul's father, Andy, stopped working to look after the boys. Two years later he met and married Elaine and they had a daughter. Paul liked Elaine and they developed a close, loving relationship.

Paul moved to middle school where an older boy repeatedly taunted him about his mother's death. Eventually Paul hit him and they both ended up in detention. He was angry and started blaming David for the death of their mother. Their previously close relationship became highly conflictual with constant arguing and fighting.

Assessment

The assessment indicated that Andy and Elaine were very concerned about Paul's changed behaviour. They had liaised with the school and the bullying stopped. Each had made a point of spending time with Paul, doing things he liked doing and encouraging him to talk about his feelings but it had not helped and Paul continued to feel angry. They decided he needed different help. The family's emotional openness, combined with their willingness to support rather than blame Paul for his behaviour, indicated the appropriateness of offering individual sessions for Paul. Andy brought Paul each week and waited while he was in the playroom.

Six sessions

Paul's first session started with exploring the playroom and brief spells of 'settling-in' activities, involving sword fighting and playing board games. He moved on to painting pictures of the family's summer holiday and talking about other families he had seen there. He described other boys he had met and the activities they had done. He was surprised how quickly the hour passed and said he was already looking forward to the next one.

During the second and third sessions he developed some sand-play in which he put fences around a pride of lions and dotted other animals around them. He removed the animals one by one until there was only a giraffe left. He said the giraffe wanted to be part of the lion family but could not because it needed to live where there were tall trees. He placed the giraffe on the higher level of the sand tray and planted a couple of trees nearby. The symbolism of being apart from and connected to his birth mother, and of his longing to be with her, was very strong. I said nothing about this and the following week he said that he has two mothers who love him, one in heaven and one here. The bully's taunts just showed how ignorant he was because he could not see what the truth really was.

Shortly after the second session David had complained about not going to the playroom because it was his mother too who had died. Although I offered separate sessions for David, Paul wanted his last two sessions with him. I thought he had achieved what he needed to and was not avoiding or resisting the work; he also wanted to restore his relationship with his brother.

David joined him for the last two sessions during which they played vigorously together and shared the playroom in an even-handed way.

Outcome

Andy and Elaine were struck by how much calmer Paul was at home and by the improvement in the brothers' relationship. Elaine said Paul had become affectionate to her again and had told her about how he had two mothers. His changed understanding of how he could have the best of both worlds touched his parents.

Six weeks later, at the follow-up visit, these improvements had stabilized. Paul, who previously had resisted any extra-curricular activities, had joined the after-school football club and earned a place on the team.

Closing thoughts

A therapeutic service is a process with benefits at every stage. From the first 'phone call to the last contact the quality of the client's emotional security is of paramount importance. It is only when the individual feels secure that, to use Bowlby's (1980) analogy, the therapeutic safari into potentially dangerous territory can begin. The relationship with the worker is a fundamental part of that secure base.

Sometimes it is enough for the client's story to be heard and responded to over the telephone – the reassurance that someone listens, understands and is there whenever the need to talk again arises may be all that is needed. Sometimes the family needs an outsider who can make it safe enough for them to be together and share their thoughts and feelings. Sometimes it is a long process of engagement during which experiences and defensive strategies are reviewed and repositioned in order for the work to be possible at all.

Families that have endured and survived the sequential crises of degenerative illness come with a host of strengths, but are often too exhausted by the process to recognize their achievements. The effectiveness of a service rests upon the ability to assess what is happening within the family, what it means to them, what resources are already available and what else is needed. Intervention combines these elements with a judgement about what change is possible and how this can best be achieved.

The challenge for practitioners is to remain open to whatever the next person may bring, recognizing that each person has had the resourcefulness and creative strength to get to that point. Our work is to acknowledge all that has been achieved so far and to see how much further we can go together.

References

Allison S, Stacey K, Dadds V *et al.* (2003). What the family brings: gathering evidence for strengths-based work. *Journal of Family Therapy* **25**:263–84.

Axline V (1989). *Play therapy.* Edinburgh: Churchill Livingstone.

Bell M (2002). Promoting children's rights through the use of relationship. *Child and Family Social Work.* **7**:1–11.

Trust circles. Spring (1998*a*) *Bereavement Care* **17**(1):14.

Drawing the boundaries. Summer (1998*b*) *Bereavement Care* **17**(2):27.

The volcano of anger. Summer (1999) *Bereavement Care* **18**(2):26.

Putting the child in the frame. Spring (2001*a*) *Bereavement Care* **20**(1):12.

Button sculpting. Summer (2001*b*) *Bereavement Care* **20**(2):29.

Bluebond-Langner M (1996). *In the shadow of illness: parents and siblings of the chronically ill child.* New Jersey: Princeton University Press.

Bowlby J (1980). *Loss: sadness and depression.* London: Pelican.

Bowlby J (1988). *A secure base – clinical applications of attachment theory.* London: Tavistock/Routledge.

Cattanach A (1993). *Play therapy with abused children.* London: Jessica Kingsley.

Dyregrov A (1995). *Grief in children—a handbook for adults.* London: Jessica Kingsley.

Edelson JL (1999). Children's witnessing of adult domestic violence. *Journal of Interpersonal Violence* **14**(8) August.

Fantuzzo JW, Paola LM, Lambert L *et al.* (1991). Effects of interpersonal violence on the psychological adjustment and competencies of young children. *Journal of Consulting and Clinical Psychology* **59**(2):258–65.

Glaser D (1995). Emotionally abusive experiences. In: P Reder, C Lucey (ed.) *Assessment of parenting: psychiatric and psychological contributions.* London: Routledge.

Gore S, Eckenrode J (1996). Context and process in research on risk and resilience. In: R Haggerty, M Sherrod, N Garmezy *et al.* (ed.) *Stress, risk and resilience in children and adolescents: process, mechanisms and interventions.* Cambridge: Cambridge University Press.

Hemmings P (1995). Communicating with children through play. In: S Smith, M Peennels (ed.) *Interventions with bereaved children.* London: Jessica Kingsley.

Hendriks J, Black D, Kaplan T (1995). *When father kills mother: guiding children through trauma and grief.* London: Routledge.

Humphreys C, Mullender A (2003). Children and domestic violence: a research review of the impact on children. *Research in Practice.*

Langrock AM, Compas BE, Keller G *et al.* (2002). Coping with the stress of parental depression: parents' reports of children's coping, emotional and behavioural problems. *Journal of Clinical Child and Adolescent Psychology* **31**(3):312–24.

Miller A (1992). *For your own good: the roots of violence in child-rearing.* London: Virago.

Nichols M, Schwartz R (ed.) (1995). *Family therapy concepts and methods.* 3rd edn. Boston, MA: Allyn & Bacon.

Radke-Yarrow M, Nottelmann E, Martinez P *et al.* (1992). Young children of affectively ill parents: a longitudinal study of psychosocial development. *Journal of American Academy of Child and Adolescent Psychiatry* **31**:1 January, pp. 68–77.

Reder P, Duncan S (1995). The meaning of the child. In: P Reder, C Lucey (ed.) *Assessment of parenting: psychiatric and psychological contributions.* London: Routledge.

Wertheimer A (1991). *A special scar.* London: Routledge.

Wilson K, Kendrick P, Ryan V (1992). *Play therapy – a non-directive approach for children and adolescents.* London: Balliere Tindall.

Yule W, Perrin S, Smith S (2000). Post-traumatic stress reactions in children and adolescents. *Post-traumatic stress disorders- concepts and therapy.* Chichester: Wiley.

Chapter 5

Therapeutic interventions

Patsy Way and Isobel Bremner

Introduction

We are members of the Candle project team at St Christopher's Hospice, described elsewhere (Chapter 8, The extended warranty by Frances Kraus). We are involved in individual, group, and family work but will give less emphasis to group work here as this is more fully described in Chapter 6 (One-off or once a term: brief interventions in groupwork by Frances Kraus).

Isobel comes from a psychodynamic background and Patsy works from a systemic family therapy tradition. Our methods are similar in that we offer a brief intervention to children and families, usually with a maximum of six sessions in very child-friendly surroundings in St Christopher's Hospice in South London. We have a playroom with art, craft, and play materials. In this chapter we will reflect on some techniques we have used and outline our thinking in making specific interventions with a particular young person or family. For convenience, Isobel describes work with adolescents and Patsy focuses on children, though we both work with both groups. Names and identifying features of children and young people we work with have been changed to protect confidentiality.

Techniques for working with bereaved children

John Burnham (1992) has made a distinction between approach, method, and technique in a piece of work, noting that counsellors might share similar approaches but have very different methods and techniques or perhaps, as in this case, come from different approaches but have similarities on methods and/or techniques. The focus in this chapter is on techniques.

We can draw on a rich heritage of professional stories, developed as theories of bereavement, to support our work and I would place my work in a narrative tradition (Gergen and Gergen 1984). I see my task as attempting to facilitate child and family in conversations that will continue at home and elsewhere and invite them to draw on their own resilience and resources to incorporate the dead person into the autobiography of their past, present, and future.

Why use play? Different techniques for different purposes

When first meeting a parent/carer or family I ask why they have chosen to access the Candle Project at this point in bereavement, sometimes very soon after the death, sometimes as long as two or three years later. I enquire about what referrers, parent/carers, and children themselves are most concerned about and the answers may be very different in each case. I also ask about what they hope for from coming. Are they perhaps assuming that, since this is a reputable organization offering a service it must be a 'Good Thing' for children or do they have particular hopes, even if not fully articulated, that they will be able to move on as a family in an area they are finding difficult? My hope is that we can begin to play and talk in a way that can continue and develop at home.

The organizational expectations are that the intervention be brief, to a maximum of five or six sessions. It is therefore crucial that the intervention and the focus of the work is clearly defined and that the techniques chosen for work with a family can engage the imagination and creative energies of both children and adults together (Lewis and Kavanagh 1995). Playful techniques are used as a language to connect with children. Thus the resources in the playroom, the hospice, and the wider world are utilized to develop helpful and strong narratives promoting resilience in children and families. These ideas are intended not as prescriptions for intervention but more as a stimulus for creative responses to engage children.

Some familiar techniques to engage children

Some techniques are well described in the literature. For example, Winston's Wish in their 'Muddles, Puddles and Sunshine' activity book (Crossley 2000) describe use of a memory box for treasures which relate to or belonged to the deceased. Similarly, I describe below my use of memory jars to enrich a child's narrative of precious memories of a dead person. Memory jars are one of many ways of using colour association to talk with a child about special memories.

Jenny's mother Wendy died nearly a year ago. She is an only child and, along with her father, is struggling to weave memories of Wendy into her new life without her. We made a memory jar using a recycled spice jar and salt coloured with chalks.

While we prepared the coloured salt Jenny described an early and joyful memory of going to the seaside with her mother before she was wheelchair bound. Jenny put blue salt in the first layer of the jar, reminding her of the sea. This was followed by yellow for the sandy beach they had picnicked on and reminded her of her peanut butter sandwiches. A layer of pink salt evoked the pink icing on the birthday cake her mother had ordered specially for her fifth birthday and mauve reminded her of Wendy's nightgown when she was ill and Jenny visited her in hospital. Jenny was able to take this jar home and place it on display for others to admire her craftwork. This allowed her choices about explaining her associations with the colours to those such as her father, grandmother, and her best friend with whom she wanted to share these private thoughts.

A range of similar colour association techniques can be used such as marbling kits. Coloured inks require no artistic talent to use and always result in an interesting and pleasing result of swirls of colour.

Learning about the family

Pearce (1994) has discussed the idea of 'stories lived' and 'stories told'. Engaging parent/carers and children in drawing a family tree together can provide a way into understanding how members of a family tell stories about themselves and their deceased relatives and also what understanding children have about events surrounding the bereavement.

Mrs F came with four children under seven years old. Their grandfather, who had lived in the family home, had been murdered in Ghana, his country of origin. He had been a very significant figure for the children as their father no longer had contact. I invited Mrs F and each child to choose a different coloured felt tip to draw up a family tree with me. Explaining that we use a circle for a girl or woman and square for boy or man, I invited children to write their names and ages. As family, friends, and pets were added to the tree in turn, children and adults elaborated on how they played a role in their lives, telling anecdotes about an aunt, her cat, her favourite food, what happened when .... All this enabled a conversation that included even the youngest in the room, allowed the children a growing confidence in working with me and gave me a view on how this family communicate together, who takes the lead, who is most listened to, and what is acceptable to say or not say.

One of the twins hesitated about drawing in his goldfish, who had died, on the family tree. The six year old used the phrase 'Lost my grandad' and was unsure where his grandfather was lost. On the way to heaven? In Ghana? This allowed opportunities to unfold the story of how grandad died, what happened to his body (including explanations that his body couldn't see, feel, or talk), the body being sent back to Ghana, the burial. We were able to look up Ghana on the map and see it was a long way away but a real place, a place the children might visit one day. We talked about funerals (using picture books) and what happens and what people do. We talked about heaven (this is a church-going family) as a different kind of place. We discussed differences between body and spirit. I was given openings for conversations in future sessions with the older girls who were left with issues of anger, guilt, forgiveness, and retribution.

Checking in: What else is happening in your life (including the good things!)

When someone dies, children's worlds may be turned upside down with a series of secondary losses. Some families will have economic stressors after a family member dies. The remaining parent/carer may be taking a new job and the family may need to move. Children may be looked after differently, families split, and young people may need to change schools.

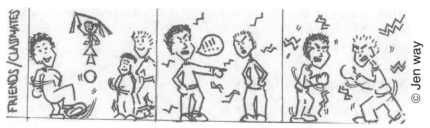

Fig. 5.1 Check in sheet: How's it going with friends and classmates?

Children and families may not be recognizing the effect of this on themselves and the way they connect with each other. I developed a 'how's it going?' sheet to address these areas (see Fig. 5.1; Check in sheet).

This can be done quickly and non-verbally at the beginning of sessions with children and families. It allows me an insight into how the child(ren) experienced the intervening time since the last meeting. It allows children to tell me more about areas I might not know or ask about, or they might think important to them but irrelevant to bereavement. It allows exploration of important experiences that may not be deemed relevant by others. Five categories address health, relationships with adults in school, parent/carers, and peers, and a general 'feelings' section. Three illustrations are offered in each section reflecting degrees of upset in a particular context. The child is invited to tick the illustration best reflecting their recent experience. If parent/carers or others in the family are present they can comment from their point of view. Children can then decide whether to tell me more about, for example, an upsetting episode at home, or keep it private. The sheet can be done in a couple of minutes and put aside or become the basis of the whole session if interesting and important stories emerge.

Sam is nine years old and without siblings. He has been trying so hard to be helpful to his mother Jane who talks about him as 'my little man', helping with cooking, washing up, and locking up the house at night as his father used to. He is confused and uncertain about his father's death six months ago when he fell on a railway line following an alcoholic binge. The school has tried hard not to worry Jane who they see as distraught and finding it hard to be available to her son. Another child taunted him in the playground with, 'Where's your dad then?' On using the check in sheet Sam said, 'it's not really about dad but...' and recounted the story of how he had reacted to the taunting by fighting because he felt upset and confused, not knowing the answer to the question. I asked questions about what was alright or not alright to ask mummy about. Jane in turn gave voice to her love and concern for Sam in spite of her sadness. We could then think about practical strategies for managing such incidents in school, inviting the support of his class teacher.

In a subsequent session we picked up on Sam's wider worries and invited him to draw a cross-section of his brain, showing the proportion of his thinking taken up with different things (see Fig. 5.2; Brain Cross-Section).

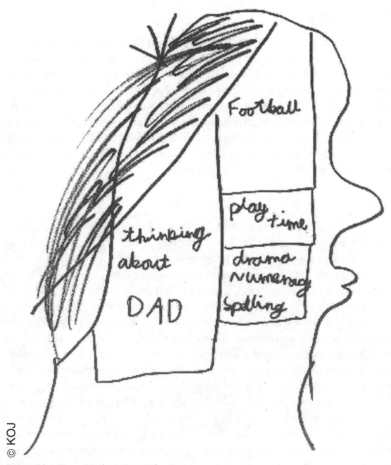

© KOJ

Fig. 5.2 Brain Cross-Section: Sam's brain

Jane was amazed at how much of his attention he showed as thoughts of his dad and worries about her health and abilities to cope. She had imagined he was rather irritatingly absent at times and showing general laziness and inattention in school. This image started a conversation that led onto discussions about what each could expect from the other. It allowed for explanations and reassurances that although she was stressed and unhappy she was not terminally ill as he feared. We explored Sam's questions about 'dad on the railway' and Jane explained in simple language about the coroner having found out all about it, like a detective, and deciding that his father had fallen under the train, probably because his brain was all muddled up from drinking the beer but that we do not know exactly what happened or why. Sam asked if his father might have done it on purpose and Jane said this was possible but she did not know. She reassured him that she and his father loved him very much and if his father had made that kind of mistake when his head was muddled from the drink, it was not to do with Sam because his father and she loved him very much.

Externalizing

We know (Rowling 2003) that 'gender can be a significant disenfranchizing issue for young males in schools' and that bereaved boys are more likely to show behaviours in school likely to lead to serious consequences and sometimes permanent exclusion. Bereaved children are often managing a series of secondary losses which may impact on their lives for a long time. Boys often react with anger and aggression when confused and upset, which then attracts an angry response. White (White and Epston 1990) developed ideas of 'externalizing' some behaviours as a technique for shifting the blame outside of the individual, particularly when it seems that one member of the family appears to carry the weight of criticism.

Junior is six years old. His teacher is complaining that, though she knows he is a bright boy, he behaves differently since his older brother died. His brother had special needs and suffered from a complex medical condition. Though there had always been concerns about his disabilities there had not been any expectation that he would die so young and suddenly. Junior's teacher, though initially very sympathetic, feels that more than a year after the death this can no longer be an excuse for Junior's isolated and angry behaviours in school, which are causing him to lose friends and his teachers to lose patience. Junior's mother, bereaved and utterly exhausted, is exasperated. At home Junior is generally helpful and caring towards her with only occasional outbursts of temper. She is having to attend frequent meetings in school about what is described as his increasingly aggressive and antisocial behaviour. She would agree with his teachers that bereavement can no longer be an excuse.

I began asking whether Junior was familiar with Roger Hargreaves' books about the 'Mr Men'. His favourite was Mr Tickle and, following a conversation with him and his mother about events in school I wondered aloud if 'Mr Angry' might have been visiting him. Would he be more likely to visit him at home or at school? In the classroom or in the playground? When his teacher was there or not? Did he visit anyone else at home or at school? Junior pointed out that there wasn't really a Mr Angry and I replied, inviting him into a playful and imaginative space, saying 'How would we know? Perhaps there is?'

Junior looked intrigued and I expanded my theme that perhaps Mr Angry might be sneaking up to him when he was most vulnerable in the classroom and inviting him to the kicking, punching, and rude behaviours that upset his classmates and teachers.

I wondered what Mr Angry might look like and Junior began to create him out of playdough using a kit that provides little plastic arms, legs, eyes, and hats while I chatted to him, asking about how Mr Angry might be affecting his life. Junior engaged playfully, answering questions such as, 'If he invites you to do these things, what are the consequences?' It got Junior himself into big trouble, upset his mother, teachers, and school friends and the only person who would enjoy it all would be Mr Angry himself. I wondered aloud if Mr Angry might not have a team of nasty characters egging him on, such as Mr Punch, Mr Temper, and Mr Not-Pay-Attention.

Junior made them all in turn in playdough and as he did so I asked him for more detail about how these characters were spoiling his life in school. I pointed out that we, of course knew that this was not the 'real' Junior, who, from previous descriptions, was very helpful and supportive of his mother. I began to wonder about a team of other characters, led by Mr Helpful, who invited Junior to behaviours that others enjoyed and admired. At the close of the session I set Junior and his mother some 'homework'. We took a Polaroid photo of him with the playdough characters, to be put on the fridge door or some other prominent place. Junior and his mum were to note down any time when they thought Mr Angry and friends were going to invite Junior into unhelpful behaviours but he managed to listen to Mr Helpful and his crew.

At the next meeting, Junior's mother reported on times she had noticed James escaping from Mr Angry, some occasions that Junior himself had not noticed until it was pointed out. Junior enjoyed explaining to me in detail how he had, with support from Mr Helpful, chosen to act differently in school also. His mother had taken a supportive classroom assistant, Mrs Jones, into their confidence and she was also helping to look out for 'escapes' from Mr Angry and company in the school playground and relaying these observations to the class teacher. I could then offer certificates and stickers to recognize these important escapes. This also enabled a conversation about when and how anger can be useful and necessary, and I could then invite Junior to think about how he experienced anger in his body and how he chose to deal with it and manage it in different situations at home and school.

In this externalizing technique White invites children to look at their behavioural choices from a position of not feeling blamed, on the premise that change is more likely to occur when one is not defending one's behaviour. Externalizing allows other, forgotten and more positive descriptions of a child to re-emerge and allows all those involved to separate the behaviours from the person. (Fig. 5.3; Mr Angry and Mr Helpful.)

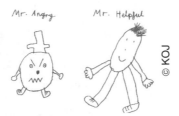

Fig. 5.3 Mr Angry and Mr Helpful

In the final session, Junior drew Mr Angry and we photocopied him in different sizes. Junior thought Mr Angry was now 'pocket sized' and manageable and might have some uses. As he got bigger, however, he was not helpful, so that an A3 sized Mr Angry would probably cause more trouble for him in school. The school assistant and his mother were then able to ask Junior how big Mr Angry was on a particular day and take their cue on how much nurturing and monitoring Junior was asking for. This enabled a supportive dialogue to begin to develop between home and school, no longer focusing on blaming Junior.

Time line

Michael White (1989) invites the bereaved to 'say hello again' to the deceased. Having mourned the loss and changes in their lives he suggests ways of working with people to bring that person into their present and future thinking. This has resonances with Tony Walter's work (1999). Children and families are sometimes uncertain of how someone who has been central in their lives can continue to be part of their present and future as well as being held in past memory. Many are afraid of memories fading and feeling that the person will then be lost forever. I have adapted ideas from White (2001) which I have presented here as a time line.

Laura is 11 and about to transfer to secondary school, losing the familiarity of a small primary setting where everyone knows her. She is the eldest of three girls and her mother died of cancer eight months ago after a long illness which began after the birth of the youngest child. Laura has been 'the little mother' during two house moves, illness, and remissions. Her father, who is attentive and concerned about her, has a new partner who is pregnant. Laura herself has just had her first period. In the next few months Laura will have a new sibling, a new caring adult, and a new school. Recently she has been bad tempered and uncharacteristically aggressive. She is usually seen as friendly, helpful, and competent, appreciated by family, friends, and teachers.

In our meeting I pulled out a roll of wallpaper and we drew two parallel lines. The bottom one was the time line on which we recorded important dates and events, from her parents' first meeting and her birth and continuing on into her future and adulthood. I asked her and her father about the qualities they valued in her and how she had developed these.

Stories emerged of patience and competence in looking after babies and her ill mother. They spoke of her drama skills in school, encouraged by her mother, her funny jokes, and dances as a little girl. She was described attending to her mother's needs for gentleness, quiet, and distraction at different stages of the illness.

We connected this (literally, with a coloured felt-tip) to events and stories that included other family members and friends, noticing how she was the same and also different from her mother. A rich story emerged of Laura's developing skills and qualities over time, nurtured by her mother and others. We projected these into the future and I asked questions such as, 'I wonder how these abilities will show in your new school? How will this ability to connect and communicate with others develop in college or university? In your first job? With your first boyfriend?'

In this way particular memories were deepened and in the process of telling and listening to these memories descriptions of Laura that connected her with her mother and others and emphasized her strengths and resourcefulness were linked with her past, present, and future. This allowed new conversations to develop around her place in her newly forming family and the way in which Laura and her abilities are valued. This included her father's new partner and the baby in her present and future and allowed her to talk about her mother with them in a way that did not invite her to feel disloyal to her memory or to new and emerging aspects of her own identity.

The last session

The last session provides an opportunity to review the work and think about changes that have happened and are hoped for, including the deceased in thinking about the past, present, and future and perhaps putting together a little book of the worksheets. Ending rituals of photographs and the gift of a little bear mark the parting but the 'extended warranty' (see Chapter 8) is offered and a child will be invited to the group day. Parents may also be encouraged to attend one of the groups.

Techniques for working with bereaved young people

Young people managing the turbulence of adolescence and grief at the same time have a lot to process. They may also be managing the pressure of secondary schooling, sexual relationships, and intense ambivalence towards their parents/carers. They are unlikely to want to see a professional and have usually arrived under duress feeling very aggrieved that anyone would think that they need help. This is the context in which much work with young people begins, so how do we make a connection and move forward in a very short space of time?

The techniques I outline below have developed out of the constraints of time and the necessity to engage very quickly with the young person as I never know whether I will see them again.

Initial contact

I start by checking that the young person knows why they are at the project and who referred them. I may read out the referral form to the young person and their parent/carer to make sure that the information is correct. I initially see the young person with the parent/carer and encourage the adult to give me quite a lot of details about their concerns in front of the young person. Sometimes this is the only intervention needed.

> I met a 13-year-old boy whose brother had died. His parents brought him in and were very concerned about him not expressing any grief about the death. The parent's telling of the story indicated that they had very different ways of coping with the death. One of them was processing their grief through a very open expression of their feelings, which the family found overwhelming. The other was managing their grief by thinking the issues through and distancing themselves from their feelings. The son was behaving like one of the parents and the concerns were primarily those of the other parent. They were able to acknowledge this and found some counselling for themselves as a couple about how to live with each other's very different ways of grieving.

When I see a young person I often draw a body outline and ask them to fill in their feelings using different colours (Heegaard 1998). I use this to establish a baseline for me in terms of what their key feelings are, to affirm that a range of feelings in response to a death is usual and to establish that words are not the only medium with which to communicate feelings. The young people I have worked with have been surprisingly open to drawing.

I used body outlines with a 15 year old who had experienced the recent death of a grandparent and was also managing the reawakening of his distress about the death of a parent. He filled in 2 outlines for me, one on his feelings about his grandparent and the other with his feelings about the parental death. I referred to them in most of the sessions checking whether they had changed, and if they had, what had helped to change them. They were a clear visual way of showing this young person that he had changed and progressed significantly in allowing himself to process feelings rather than just desperately holding onto them hoping they would go away.

Affirming the grief reaction of the young person

Many young people are referred on the basis that they do not cry about the death. It is crucial that the young person and their parent/carer know that this is not unusual. Young people may be too unsettled and fearful to cry, especially in front of another person. Lewis (1966) writes, 'No one ever told me that grief felt so like fear'. Young people are already managing a lot of fear as they experience adolescence; to compound this with the anxiety that grief may produce can be quite overwhelming. To cry you need to feel reasonably safe and secure. Christ's (2000) research is very interesting in looking at the differences between early (12–14) and middle (15–17) adolescence. Early adolescents can have moments of acute grief and long periods of not expressing their grief. Again this needs to be affirmed and normalized. The sense that however you feel or are expressing your grief is right for you at that moment is crucial in setting up an atmosphere of trust and developing a relationship. Many young people believe they are not doing it right and are worrying about themselves or believing that they are uncaring, unloving, or pathetic. They are negatively reframing their reactions to the death. I try to normalize this along the lines of it is very usual to be intensely critical of oneself following the death of someone close to you. I sometimes explain it as the 'catch 22' or double bind of grief.

A young woman believed that she was pathetic and useless because she cried at school and felt overwhelmed whenever she was reminded that her mother was dead. I helped her to reframe this by thinking of herself as someone who was sad because she loved and missed her mother.

At Candle we give young people the Candle leaflets 'Someone close to you has died' (2002) and 'Someone has died suddenly' (1999) to affirm the types of reactions they may have. Younger adolescents also like the little concertina leaflets 'A Pocket Book For Teenagers' and the 'Is This Normal?' poster from Bereavement Care in Staffordshire (Jordan and Rodway 1997a, b).

Affirming the difference

Young people frequently talk about how different they feel to their peers since the death. Often they do not know other young people who are bereaved. Their whole world perspective changes when someone close to them has died. They can be irritated with the usual concerns of adolescence, finding over dramatic references from other teenagers about wishing their parents were dead very offensive. They may feel the politics of the playground are trivial. They often need help with how to talk to their peers about the death and to be encouraged to verbalize their distress rather than act it out.

They need to know that they are now seeing the world from a unique and different standpoint. This is out of the ordinary and is particularly hard on them because of their youth. However there are now valuable qualities about themselves that they would not have found if they had not experienced this death. I use the example of a house with rooms that you never knew existed. These rooms may initially be dark but with some exploration they may discover gifts, strengths, and sides to themselves that they never knew existed. They can also, should they wish to, shut the doors of these rooms and return to ordinary adolescence.

A young woman whose father had died, insisted she was different since his death and wanted to return to her old self. She realized that her new compassion and understanding for other troubled young people was a consequence of the death of her father and was something to be valued. Once she had accepted this she also began to find her old self again.

Open and transparent counselling

One of the aims of my work is to enable the young person to learn how to self manage their grief. The significant event of the death of someone close to them is never going to go away. Their reaction to the death is of value and needs to be responded to with concern and interest. They can learn to manage and if necessary change this reaction.

The way that I convey this is by being open about the process that goes on inside me as I do the work in terms of my different reactions to them, my choices about the work we are to do, and also my own struggle with emotion or not usually spoken about thoughts. Obviously I do this with an awareness of the context but I do it as genuinely as I can. The aim being to model:

- The usefulness of transparency about inner conflict when working out what to do;
- The value of speaking out loud about feelings and thoughts even if anxiety provoking;
- The possible range of feelings that are around when working on grief; the lack of magic answers to the big issues in life like the death of someone;
- The importance of valuing inner uncertainty.

A young person whose father had died was very worried because he kept 'seeing' his father. I was open about my own uncertainty about what this was about and wondered out loud; was it a ghost or was the young person hallucinating? He acknowledged that he had thought about both explanations and both frightened him. I reassured him that bereaved people often think that they hear or 'see' the person who died. We explored his fears and the possible causes of either option. The hallucinations/ghost stopped after this session.

Being open about my feelings in response to being told about the death and not suppressing tears, fear or anger models the safe expression of feelings. This needs to be done in a way which also coveys a capacity to continue to be professional. Some young people need reassurance that they are not a burden or that their feelings are not destructive, they may previously have not expressed their grief to adults because of their fear of overwhelming them. It is vital to show the young person that it is possible to be okay and to have very powerful feelings.

Concern about wellbeing of parent/carer

It is reasonable for young people to be concerned about their parent/carer's wellbeing. The ability of their adult carer to manage their caring role as well as their own grief has a large impact on the young person's well being (Christ 2000). However young people's expression of this concern may not be straightforward. They may act out their anxieties by being angry with the adult for expressing sadness, for example. Young people may come to counselling because of this concern about their adult carer and may need to talk about their fears and help to address them with the adult.

Young people maybe very worried about their carer's mental or physical health or their financial situation. I ask for permission to share this worry with the adult concerned and advise on where they can get support if the anxiety is a valid one or encourage the adult to offer reassurance if it is not.

A young man I have been working with was worried about his parent running up a huge credit card bill and appearing to be continuing to spend. The parent had not appreciated how concerned her son was and took steps to manage this debt.

As with adults and younger children many bereaved young people might have been sensitized to the possibility that any of those who they care about can die. They may be less likely to articulate their anxiety about this because part of their developmental task as adolescents is to separate from their parent or carer. They may want to avoid acknowledging dependency or to show that they care about their parent or carer. Parents and carers may need to be encouraged to broach this subject and make open and clear arrangements for the care of the young person in the event of their death.

Clarifying and gathering information

A part of the process of grieving is about facing the reality of what has happened and then managing our feelings about that reality (Worden 1991). Often young people do not know what has happened, or are muddled about significant events. This may be because no one has told them or because they did not want to hear at the time. Sometimes the death may have happened when they were younger and no one has since given them further more age appropriate information.

The process of information gathering may be an important part of the intervention with the young person. Often the information that I am muddled about will give me a clue about the things that need sorting out for the young person. I have used family trees and life event chronologies to help clarify what is really significant to the young person.

> A young woman whose mother had died only a year previously, talked about her as if she had died at least 3 years earlier. To try and resolve this I worked with the young woman on her life story and her family tree. I wrote out her life history as she described it to me and drew a geneogram of her family. We worked out that the significant issue for this young person was not actually the death but the very serious stroke her mother had had about 3 years earlier and the subsequent life changes and loss of the parent she had known. The young person had not received any therapeutic help at this time and was still living with powerful mixed feelings about her incapacitated mother and the relief she felt when she died. Those around her had assumed the issue was the death of her mother, whereas the young person's most burdensome feelings were guilt about the arguments she had had with her, and her lack of warm feelings towards her mother following the stroke.

If the death has been traumatic the young person may not have been given all the information out of an adult concern to protect them from the horrors of the world. This may leave the young person with a sense of being excluded and not valued by the adults who care for them. The Childhood Bereavement Network video (2002) shows young people expressing very clearly and movingly how important it is to them to be included, when important information is being shared.

> I met with a young person whose father committed suicide 8 years previously and whose feelings had been reawakened by the subsequent death of another more distant relative. She knew that there was a note written by her father and that her mother had a copy and she wanted to see the note. I encouraged her to ask her mother to see it and we then had a meeting with her mother at which she shared more information about the mode of death, which the young person had not known about. The family then contacted the coroner's officer and found out further details. This helped allay a longstanding fear of the young person that her father had committed suicide because of something she had done. The information from the inquest, the witness statements, and the suicide note all made it clear that this man committed suicide for other reasons and that he had loved his children even though he had not seen them for a number of years prior to the death.

Sometimes the young person may not have information about the death because the adults do not have it either and part of the work is to enable the adults to find out any information that is available. It is easy to be so overwhelmed by the enormity of a death that we feel helpless and unable to be proactive. It can be helpful for the parent/carer concerned to do some information finding as this gives them a sense of being in control and in alliance with both the young person and the counsellor. They may need support to do this and some pointers about how to do it.

A 15-year-old girl had been told by a stranger that her father had died. Her mother had been separated from her father for most of this young person's life and had no contact with the father's family. She needed to find out the details of the death, so that the young person could deal with these instead of continuing to be in a state of uncertainty. The daughter had felt unable to ask her mother for fear of upsetting her. The mother needed to overcome her own feelings about this man she had left many years earlier. I did a piece of work with her about acknowledging her distress and her daughter's need for information. She made contact with the paternal extended family and her daughter was hugely appreciative about finding a side to her family she had never really known before as well as finding out details about her father.

The use of bereavement models, writings, and research

Young people who come for bereavement counselling need help to make sense of their experience following the death. Developmentally they have the cognitive maturity to grasp sophisticated concepts and generally respond well to being given information about research, models, and theories.

One model to which some young people respond positively is Stroebe's dual process model (Stroebe 1999). It is useful because it is a good visual tool and because it is a reassuring description of the grieving process. Christ's research (Christ 2000) indicates that early adolescents move between infrequent strong grief reactions and then long periods of carrying on as if nothing has changed. The dual process model describes how usual this is and also how helpful it is to have times where we focus on grief and times where we focus on other issues and the future. I have used this model when working with teenagers of all ages. I have drawn it and explained it to a young woman who was managing the sudden death of her best friend. It helped her to feel it was acceptable to be excited about going to university.

To my surprise I have found that CS Lewis' book (1966) about his grief when his wife died was felt to be really helpful by an older teenager who liked Lewis' description of the many internal conflicts she herself was feeling about her grief.

Colin Murray Parkes' (1972) work is very helpful as a straightforward description of the wide range of feelings that anyone may have following the death of someone close to them. Young people may need some basic education about these feelings. It can also be helpful to remind young people that many adults have explored and written about the mysteries and workings of grief without ever reaching a definitive answer.

However what we do know is that it can have a bigger impact than we ever expected and that it can be survived well.

Working with a lack of response

Young people will rarely give you or the work you are doing with them a warm positive response. As a professional it is vital to remember that a lack of enthusiasm about the work we are doing with them is not an indication of the impact we are having. If the young person turns up for sessions it probably means they feel hopeful about the work being fruitful. Even if they do not come this does not mean that they do not think the work is useful, it may just be that they cannot do the work at that time. They may come back later and it is worth giving the young person your contact details early on for this reason.

Endings

The importance of an acknowledged ending cannot be underestimated. At the last session with a young person I will go through my notes and the body drawings with the young person present to remind them of the work we have done, the changes that have happened, and to give them feedback about how they have been, their strengths, and appreciations that I have of them. I will ask them to tell me the best thing about our work together and the most difficult thing. I will also help them think about the future and what they will do when they reach a bad patch. I will offer them the group for young people that we run and remind them that they can always re-refer themselves. I will also inform them of any local counselling services they could access in the future.

If they do not attend a last session, I will phone or write with a similar agenda to the above and I take care to give them some positive feedback and remind them they can come back.

Conclusion

We have offered our experience of working in a particular context and within a limited time frame with children, young people, and families. We have outlined how our approaches influence the work and hope to have conveyed key issues of connecting quickly with children and young people in ways that make sense of their experience, using a variety of techniques.

We wish to emphasize that we prioritize building alliances with our clients whether they be individual young people or whole families. We do this by focusing on their concerns and also reminding them of their strengths and highlighting how well they have survived thus far.

Sometimes our families arrive with a belief that a death will disable them forever unless they can learn to 'get over it'. Our view is that young people and families will have gained skills and abilities they may never have learned otherwise and may not yet have recognized. Our hope is that irrespective of the techniques chosen the work can support the creativity of families and young people in adjusting to a new future.

References

Burnham J (1992). Approach, method, technique: making distinctions and creating connections. *Human Systems* **3**(1):3–26.

Childhood Bereavement Network Video (2002). *A death in the lives of....* London: National Children's Bureau.

Christ G (2000). *Healing children's grief: surviving a parent's death from cancer.* Oxford: Oxford University Press.

Crossley D (2000). *Muddles, puddles and sunshine activity book.* Gloucester: Winston's Wish/ Hawthorn Press.

Gergen MM, Gergen KJ (1984). The social construction of narrative accounts. In: KJ Gergen, MM Gergen (ed.). *Historical social psychology.* Hillsdale, NJ: Lawrence Erlbaum Associates.

Heegaard M (1988). *When someone very special dies: children can learn to cope with grief.* Minneapolis, MN: Woodland Press.

Jordan G, Rodway K (1997a). *A pocket book for teenagers.* Staffordshire Bereavement Care.

Jordan G, Rodway K (1997b). *Is this normal?* Staffordshire Bereavement Care.

Lewis CS (1966). *A grief observed.* London: Faber and Faber Ltd.

Lewis P, Kavanagh C (1995). Play as dialogue, giving voice to the child in family therapy. *Human Systems* **6**(3–4):227–41.

Parkes CM (1972). *Bereavement: studies of grief in adult life.* New York: International Universities Press.

Pearce WB (1994). *Interpersonal communication: making social worlds.* New York: Harper Collins.

Rowling L (2003). *Grief in school communities: effective support strategies.* Oxford: Oxford University Press.

St Christopher's Candle Project (1999). *Someone has died suddenly.* London: St Christopher's Hospice.

St Christopher's Candle Project (2002). *Someone close to you has died.* London: St Christopher's Hospice.

Stroebe M (1999). The dual process model of coping with bereavement: rationale and description. *Death Studies 99* **23**(3):197–224.

Walters T (1999). *On bereavement: the culture of grief.* Oxford: Oxford University Press.

White M (1989). Saying hullo again: the incorporation of the lost relationship in the resolution of grief. In: M White (ed.) *Selected Papers.* Adelaide: Dulwich Centre Publications.

White M, Epston D (1990). Externalizing of the problem. In: M White (ed.) *Narrative means to therapeutic ends.* Norton, pp. 38–76.

White M (2001). Delight and the unexpected. Workshop held at School of Oriental and African Studies, University of London 14.6.01-15.6.01, offered by the Brief Therapy Practice.

Worden JW (1991). *Grief counselling and grief therapy: a handbook for the mental health practitioner,* 2nd edn. New York: Springer.

Chapter 6

One-off or once a term: brief interventions in groupwork

Frances Kraus

A group experience has significant value for bereaved children. Many children find bereavement very isolating, as they may not know of another bereaved child in their school or community, and may believe that their situation is unique. Children who are at school spend much of their time in groups, and are familiar with engaging in activities and discussions in that setting. There are increased opportunities for peer support and social learning available in a group setting, and the wider psychotherapeutic value of group experiences is well evidenced (Yalom 1975). The mapping exercise for the Childhood Bereavement Network carried out in 2002 showed that of the 47 open access bereavement services for children that had responded to the questionnaire, 33 offered group activities or support to children and 35 to parents and carers (Childhood Bereavement Network 2002).

There are many ways of structuring groups for bereaved children, but much of the literature has focused on regular on-going small groups with a closed membership meeting for a fixed number of between 6 and 12 sessions usually on a weekly basis, which may reflect the origins of therapeutic groupwork within the psychoanalytic tradition (Lohnes and Kalter 1994; Smith and Pennells 1995; Kirk and McManus 2002; Pfeffer *et al.* 2002). Another model is that of the residential weekend camp, with an emphasis on grief support rather than grief therapy, and accepting referrals for all bereaved children and families within the context of a non-pathologizing service (Stokes 2004). The programme at Candle has developed in a form that takes elements from both of these programmes, adapted and adjusted to suit the project's client group, geographical location, and resources. In this chapter, I intend to look at why we have chosen the programme we have, what it consists of, the issues that have arisen for us and some of the ways that we have tried to address them to date.

The agency

The Candle project offers short-term bereavement focused counselling to children, young people and families in the South East London area. The project was developed as an extension of the support that St Christopher's Hospice had provided for many years to patients' families, and extended this to offer an open access service to all children, young people and families in the area. The overwhelming majority of the children who come to Candle have been bereaved by a sudden and often traumatic death such as a road traffic collision, sudden illness such as a stroke or heart attack, suicide, or murder. The project aims to address the needs of bereaved children and families through the provision of individual and group support, delivered by professional paid staff and volunteers.

Development of Candle service

The Candle project began in 1998 with one full time staff member and one part time sessional worker. Families and children were seen for individual sessions in the office/playroom by these two staff members. Both had been hospice social workers with extensive experience of bereavement through terminal illness, but less experience of working with families bereaved through a sudden death. About 75% of the referrals to Candle in the first year and for all subsequent years have been for families bereaved by a sudden and often traumatic death. The decision was made to involve volunteers with the groupwork activities, but not in the delivery of the individual sessions for children and families. The groupwork programme could not start until volunteers were recruited, trained and ready, and we had seen sufficient numbers of children to make up a viable group. This necessary delay allowed time for the staff team to increase their expertise and confidence about working with these families.

There was an operational consideration to the decision to rely on professionals to deliver the core service. As the project leader and as the only full time staff member of the project, I felt that to engage volunteers to provide the direct work with the children and families would be too risky and too costly for the limited staff resources available. I had experience of a bereavement service provided by volunteers (St Christopher's Hospice), and was aware of the importance of the extensive individual and group supervision and consultation necessary to support the volunteers and deliver a high quality and reliable service. I reasoned that recruiting, checking, training, supervising, managing, and providing on-going support to a volunteer group to deliver individual work would not save on staff resources for service delivery, and this belief became stronger as I gained more experience of the complex nature of many of the bereavements and of the frequent need for liaison work with other professionals. The practicalities of supporting a volunteer through the demands of liaison with schools, health care professionals, and social services, and referrals on to other agencies, would, I felt be very time consuming for the paid staff members. Accordingly, Candle followed the model of professional service delivery for individual work. I am aware that other services have developed very successfully using volunteers to provide direct work (see Chapter 10) and that this decision might have been influenced by my need for control, but I needed to find ways to minimize my levels of anxiety as the leader of a new project. Candle operates a structure that uses the services of volunteers to provide group experiences for the children, under the supervision of a staff member, which enables volunteer involvement and limits their responsibility.

The groupwork model used in the Candle project is based on that operated by St Christopher's Hospice bereavement service for several years. This model was a one-off meeting at a weekend with an activity based format for children aged 8–12 years, as described by Baulkwill and Wood (1995). Groupwork has developed as the Candle project has grown, and we now have several different types of groups on offer at weekends or in the evenings, some of which are one-off and some are on-going, but on a limited basis only; three times a year during the school terms.

The groupwork programme at Candle

Groupwork was included in the plans for the Candle project from the outset and the staff team had skills, experience, and training in working with groups of adults and children, both from the experience in the hospice and elsewhere. As with the individual and family work, the way groupwork has been developed and delivered has been pragmatic and resource driven. Candle has a small staff team, consisting currently (2003), of two permanent paid staff including myself both working four days per week each, one paid staff member on two days per week and a sessional worker who contributes between a half and one day per week solely to activities connected to the groupwork programme. In addition to this we have 21 trained groupwork volunteers. There are four strands to the work of the project; the provision of individual and family counselling, the telephone advice and consultancy service, the provision of training and resources for professionals and families, and the groupwork programme.

Why choose to hold one-off groups?

The families we work with often find it hard to commit themselves to regular attendance, and our experience is that they sometimes fail their appointments for a variety of reasons; the many childhood illnesses all children are prone to, the extra stresses for bereaved children (Lloyd-Williams *et al.* 1998), and the difficulties for bereaved parents who are adjusting to their new practical and emotional responsibilities. One parent I worked with explained it to me metaphorically as follows, 'Sharon (his wife), was always the "driver", she made all the decisions, and I was just the passenger, and now I have to get used to being the driver for the whole family as well as missing her.' Bereaved parents or carers have to adjust to a new role as the sole carer and earner, and this places obvious limitations on their capacity to attend regular appointments.

It is possible to be flexible and accommodate individual families, but groups are different. They require intensive planning and preparation, and the date, once set, cannot be changed easily. In addition, the therapeutic value of an on-going weekly or fortnightly group with the expectation of regular commitment is compromised if members are unable to attend regularly. There is a widespread belief that groups are a 'good thing', supported by the literature and the number of bereavement services that offer groups, but we still find it quite hard to persuade families to attend, and some refuse altogether. Some children and families have difficulty meeting new people, some feel that their needs have been met by the individual work, some, as with some families bereaved of a child, feel that the group will not meet their specific needs, and for others the timing of the invitation comes when they no longer want to focus on the bereavement. Families who are uncertain have often responded positively to an invitation to a one-off event, with no requirement for further attendance, but even so, approximately twice the number of children need to be invited to ensure a group day attendance of about 12 children. In addition to these factors, there are the groups of children and families, those bereaved by suicide and with younger children, who we exclude from the standard groupwork programme for reasons given later. We now run two children's group days per year in spring and autumn.

Children's days: aims and structure

The aims of the group days are given on a flyer to parents:

> To give children a chance to meet other children in the same situation as themselves. Grief can be a very isolating experience.

> To help children learn new ways to express their feelings about what happened, and give them a chance to do so.

> To provide an opportunity for children to ask questions and share some of their memories about the person who has died.

> To offer parents and carers an opportunity to meet others in the same situation in a separate group.

> To provide children with an opportunity to have some fun and enjoy themselves.

The most important aim is listed first, and cannot be met by individual work. It is the main selling point for the group days, and the one most appreciated by the children who give a feedback to us. The next two aims can also be addressed through individual work, but a wider dimension is introduced when feelings are expressed and questions asked in a group. The mention of parents and carers emphasizes the Candle project's commitment to working with families and to offering parents the same opportunity to meet as children, and the last aim underlines the need for bereaved children and families to have a break from grief, and also places the group days outside of an expressly 'therapeutic' context. One eight year old boy wrote on his evaluation that he enjoyed 'the counselling tea party'. Very clear aims have been invaluable. They have grounded us in reality and reminded us of our limitations, which has been very helpful at times when the pressure has been on to over-extend the service in a field of scarce resources. The range of groups has developed as the team has grown in confidence and in size, and as we have responded to different groups of bereaved parents or children, always working to the aims as given above. The project began in 1998 by offering group days to children from 6–12 years, with a separate group for parents as part of the day. This was building on our experience with the St Christopher's bereavement service, starting with a model we knew well and that had worked for us. We extended this a year later to offer a group experience to young people aged 13–16 years, and after experiencing poor attendance holding these at weekends moved them to a weekday evening (Childhood Bereavement Network Video 2002).

The self-help group for parents evolved as described in Chapter 16. We review our groupwork provision regularly, and aim to try and meet the needs of the children and families that we exclude from the standard provision if we are able to by offering them a tailor-made group experience. For example, we offered a one-off specialist group for families bereaved by suicide, who are excluded from the regular children's days, and experimented with one for families with children aged 5–7 years, at the same time as we raised the lower age for the regular children's days from 6 to 8 years. We now run a regular monthly open bereavement group for newly bereaved parents, which offers support to those who are not yet able to cope with the looser structure and focus of the self-help parent carers group. A mixture of standard and specialist groups allows us to respond to 'excluded groups' and is interesting and rewarding for both staff and volunteers.

One-off groups

Children's days

A balance has to be held between accessibility, availability, and safety, as we are working with a vulnerable group of clients. These are important factors for any group, but are crucial with a one-off experience, as there is only one opportunity to get it right. The experience must be positive for the children and families as there is no time within the group day to address the issues that may arise if it were to be experienced as negative. The day is very clearly structured and led by the staff and volunteers, and staffing levels are set high to ensure that children do not get 'missed' as there will be little opportunity to address this later.

Open access

We aim to be as open as possible within our parameters, which are age range, geography, and type of death. We offer the group to families from other bereavement services within or outside our immediate area of South East London, but they do need to attend for an assessment/introduction first. That meeting is to find out what their support systems are, as we will not be able to give an on-going service to a family who live outside our catchment area, and to encourage attendance by showing them around so that they will not feel so strange when they come to the day. A few families from other services or from parts of London with no access to groups have taken up the offer.

Age range

We have found that children between the ages of 8–12 are most able to benefit from the structure of the Saturday group sessions, as they are mature enough to manage meeting a group of strange adults and children and to engage in and benefit from the range of activities provided. In our experience, children aged under 7–8 years sometimes found the separation from their parent for the five hour 'day' very difficult, and were sometimes unable to engage in the group discussions as they required more individual attention. Team members also felt that the younger children were unable to understand fully the ideas behind some of the exercises and activities, and to make the links between an activity and the purpose behind it. These factors restricted the value of the group experience for all the members. The literature on children's understanding of death suggests that most children would have reached a full understanding by 8–10 years old (Kane 1979; Lansdowne and Benjamin 1985), and it follows that this group will be able to benefit more from a group day focusing on bereavement. However, our belief in the value for all bereaved children of an opportunity to meet others in the same situation later led us to offer a group for families with younger children.

Children bereaved by suicide

We do not offer the standard group day to children bereaved by suicide or those where the death is of a similarly traumatic nature, as with certain types of murder. The latter are rare, but the families bereaved by suicide form a small but significant minority of our referrals.

The impact of hearing about a death by suicide or murder on the other members of the group is more than we feel we can manage in a one-off meeting. There is the risk that other group members might feel overwhelmed by the stories, and defend against this by creating a distance between themselves and those bereaved by suicide. There are likely to be more unanswered and unanswerable questions, and more issues of blame, responsibility, and guilt. There are often major issues for these families about the legal process that directly impact on their bereavement, and further separate them from other bereaved families in the group who do not have the same experience. As the numbers we deal with are quite small, the child and their parent or carer might be the only one in the group bereaved by suicide, and might therefore feel more rather than less isolated by that experience.

For these reasons we have excluded children and families from our standard group days, but have attempted to meet their need for a group experience through a separate provision. The exclusion does not apply to the young people's evenings, where the decision is made on an individual basis about each young person's suitability for the group.

Structure of the days

The emphasis is on activity and meeting others rather than on therapy. The approach is person centred, rather than psychodynamic. This increases the safety, as we are not aiming to take therapeutic risks, and also the accessibility, as some of our families would be reluctant to engage in anything that was labelled therapeutic. Children and parents are given a feedback form at the end of the day, which they take with them and return to us.

The shape of the day is designed to bring together a group of children who do not know each other to work on the issue that they all have in common, and leave them in a safe place to return to their parents or carers at the end. Activities vary from group to group, and examples of activities and exercises have been described in the literature, so I will not go into detail here (Dwivedi 1993; Webb 1993; Smith and Pennells 1995; Stokes 2004). The morning session starts with group introductions, and group rules, followed by exercises designed to help the children get to know each other and to facilitate openness and sharing of experience. The session with the doctor that follows provides an important opportunity for the children who have not had a chance to ask questions about topics such as the causes of death, diseases, and what happens to people when they die (Thompson and Payne 2000). Children learn from the answers to their own questions and those of others. This session is particularly important for the children bereaved by a sudden death, who have often had no opportunity to find out this information before coming to the project. At a recent group day, six out of sixteen children had experienced a father dying from a heart attack. The careful explanation of what that is and that nothing actually attacked their parent was reassuring even for those who had already heard it, but were able this time to identify with other children in the same situation. A short lunch break is followed by a treasure hunt to encourage the children to go outside for a while and use up some energy. The afternoon begins with a session led by the sessional music therapist which facilitates the expression of feelings. This often engages children who have remained outside the group for some reason. An example is of one nine year old, who had spent the morning on the fringes of all the action. He sat himself next to the music therapist when she brought out the instruments and became totally involved with the activity, which was expressing different feelings using instruments. After the session he told us 'I did "sad". It was the best'. This is followed by more intense sessions of talking through memories and feelings and a candle lighting ritual, and the day ends with another ritual to say goodbye to each other. Parents and carers are offered a separate facilitated group in the morning, and sometimes stay together informally until it is time to rejoin their children.

The adult–child ratio is very high, often almost one to one, to ensure that no child is missed if distressed and that disruptive behaviour can be contained so that it does not affect the group process. The activities are structured and staffed to allow children to engage at the level that feels comfortable to them. For instance, one child may choose to make a memory jar from coloured salts that looks very pretty but contains few actual memories. The experience of making the jar, with the help of an adult who is giving him concentrated attention and interest, validates the memories he does have, and increases his self esteem. Another child may spend a lot more time in the activity talking to the adult about his memories and the feelings they bring up, and a third child may be able to extend this to share his memory jar with other children in the group. To achieve the delicate balance between activity and therapy, all team members, both staff and volunteers, need to agree on aims, and be consistent in their approach to the day. Candle staff make the initial plans for the day, and coordinate the referrals, and then meet with the volunteers, who will do much of the preparation, a few days before the group date to brief them on the children who will be coming and allocate responsibilities. At the end of the day there is a quick debrief for any urgent issues, and the volunteers also attend an evening supervision session with the staff a few days after the group day. Staff receive separate supervision with the project leader following that. Supervision is considered further later in the chapter.

Issues

Our stated aims are met according to the feedback forms we receive from children and parents, and the comments from children when they speak to us directly. The opportunity to meet other children is much appreciated. If a group of children work really well together, it is hard to say goodbye to them and to all the opportunities there could have been for them to do more together. If children are disruptive or pose problems, they have to be given a lot of one to one attention in order to preserve the experience for others in the group, a situation that could be managed by peer pressure in an on-going group. There are some children who are unable to engage in the group day and whose behaviour makes it very difficult for others, even with close attention from the team. The desire to be as inclusive as possible has to be balanced with the restrictions necessary for a one-off experience, and we do not always get it right. Sometimes the group as a whole struggles with the balance between the therapeutic and activity elements, and we occasionally receive thank you notes from parents for the 'funday.' This may be as a result of feedback from the child, as most of the forms returned by children emphasize their enjoyment of the 'fun' activities, e.g. the treasure hunt above the more therapeutic ones.

Group experiences for the children and families excluded from the above days have followed the same basic structure but have added elements to suit the client group.

Families Bereaved By Suicide

The decision to exclude children bereaved by suicide from the children's days was difficult for a project with an ethos of inclusivity. (One practitioner states that these children are unsuited to a group intervention [Webb 1993], although I believe her to mean a group intervention on its own with no accompanying individual work). A recent comparison study found that a ten session group intervention, focusing on reactions and on strengthening coping skills for families bereaved by suicide, reduced the children's levels of psychosocial distress (Pfeffer *et al.* 2002). The reason given by Webb is the need of these children for more in-depth individual exploration of their idiosyncratic feelings, which is better managed in individual work. This has validity but does not address the very powerful feelings of isolation and stigma felt by many of these children and their parents, and we were determined to offer them the same group opportunity as soon as we were able to. The numbers of children we meet with bereaved by suicide are quite small (about 10–12 per year). It therefore follows that we have to wait some time for sufficient numbers to offer a group, and then face the possibility that some families will have moved on in their lives and will no longer be interested. The first group worked with children aged 8–12 years, and offered a separate group for parents that ran concurrently. Young people bereaved by suicide are given an invitation to the young peoples' group, if the team member who is working with them believes that they and the group will be able to cope with the issues that may arise. The young people have so far displayed great sophistication when dealing with this particular bereavement.

Structure

The day was basically structured in the same way as the children's days, with a few differences. The session of questions to the doctor focused on questions about suicide, and was provided by a local child psychiatrist with close links to the project, who also spent time with the parents at lunchtime to talk to them about their children's issues. We introduced one new exercise to allow expression of difficult as well as good memories. One child commented that it was the first time that he had been able to tell other children about what had happened, as he knew they would understand. The parent's group also lasted for the whole day rather than the morning only, which was greatly appreciated by the small group who attended.

Issues

These were both practical and therapeutic. On the practical side, it was difficult to engage enough families with the group. One family who had been waiting for some time were in foster care at the time of the group, and the carers had made other arrangements for them which they did not want to alter. Another parent changed her mind at the last minute as she received another invitation, but did allow her child to attend with another relative, who did not stay for the carer's group.

The families' ambivalent responses were in contrast to the professional anxiety experienced by members of the team, who were very aware of the extra stresses on these families and their vulnerabilities. This led to a shift in focus to risk assessment and an initial proposal for a group structured on more therapeutic lines. This was not congruent with a project which wishes to avoid pathologizing bereavement, and was later dropped.

Day for parents/carers and children aged 5–7 years

Although younger children were unable to understand some of the aims of the activities in the children's days, those who had attended had always enjoyed meeting other children in the same situation as themselves. Their parents and carers had also told us how helpful they found the days, and some of them have become members of the parent/carers group (see Chapter 16). The team therefore decided to offer a group day to families with younger children, and to work with families staying together for the whole day, with a lunchtime session for parents and children separately. The reasoning behind this decision was our experiences with children of this age, which led us to feel that the day would be more successful if we focused on the family unit rather than attempting to separate often reluctant children from their carers.

Structure

The 'day' was shorter than our usual children's days, and ran from 11 am–2 pm, by which time the children were clearly very tired. Children and carers stayed together apart from at lunchtime, when we offered the carers a separate group session over lunch while staff and volunteers took care of the children. Even then, one child would not be separated from his mother, who stayed and ate with the children. Some of the more concrete activities from the children's days were included, but the most successful ones, in terms of engaging the children's attention, were new for this group; meeting Bertie, a lifesize hand puppet of a dog, and listening to a story. Bertie talked to the children about his feelings after someone close to him died, and we chose to read aloud from one of the illustrated stories with a bereavement theme.

Issues

Staff and volunteers felt the most positive aspect of the day was the way carers and children were able to share their experiences and feelings. At times this was difficult for some of the team, who found it hard to work with the children and carers together rather than directly with the child as in the regular groups, and the day produced some valuable exploration of attitudes to parenting in the supervision session. One volunteer commented on the difficulty for her in standing back when she felt a parent was being controlling or interfering with their child's experience. The most powerful element for me as one of the workers on the day was the strong presence of the dead parent. The room felt much more full than would be expected with a small group, and seeing the children with their surviving parents or carers made me very conscious of the ghosts in the room, of the missing person in the family group, which I have not felt in other children's days.

Once a term provision

Young People's Evenings

This open group is held once a term, for young people aged 12–16 years. The young people requested more sessions after the first meeting, and the team felt that it was appropriate to respond. The reasons for our positive response to their request were a mixture of the philosophical and the practical.

◆ Younger children who attend the project are able to meet on an on-going basis if their parent comes to the parent/carers groups where child care is provided. Although these sessions are based solely around crafts and activities, all the children are aware of their commonality, and build up relationships. Young people aged 13–16 did not usually attend these sessions, as they do not wish or require child care, so it appeared consistent to offer them a chance to meet more than once.

◆ The group does not require as high an adult/child ratio as the children's days, as there is less need for a detailed and directive structure, and fewer planned activities. The activities are a means of initiating conversations between the members, who talk very readily to each other after a short time. This is in contrast to the children's days, where much more direction is needed in activities to encourage the members to talk to each other rather than to the group leaders. Staffing levels are an important factor for a small team with many other responsibilities. We could not justify running three groups a year for young people if the work involved detracted attention from the other aims of the project.

◆ It had been difficult for our service to find a group structure that worked for young people, and we had experienced several false starts. It is hard to summon up enthusiasm for a prospective group in members staff or volunteers if the last one was cancelled because there were not enough young people to make it viable. We felt that a core group of members would help to make this more certain. Young people are encouraged to attend a group if they are reassured that there will be others there in a similar situation. Some general information can also be shared with prospective members to encourage them to attend. We might say something like 'there will be a couple of other young people coming who have lost a dad, and theirs were also sudden deaths. One is your age, the other is a bit younger.' This avoids breaking confidentiality, but makes the group sound less anonymous and impersonal, and a more attractive prospect to attend. We were also considering the different needs for peer group contact that young people have, and the greater relative importance of opportunities to form relationships with others in the same situation (Childhood Bereavement Network Video 2002).

Structure

The group evenings are for young people aged 12–16 years, but we are flexible around the age parameters, and a mature 11-year-old will be invited if they have begun their secondary education. We now have a small number of 17 year olds, and have developed a policy around leaving. As with the children's days, we accept referrals from other bereavement services. About 9–12 young people attend each session.

These evenings begin at 6:30 pm with introductory exercises in small groups of four or five consisting of both old and new group members and staff, carefully matched for age and gender. Where possible for the introductory exercise we also try to place the new members in a group with at least one other young person with a similar loss. The young people are given a theme to discuss or work on in these groups. Creative therapies are used to offer young people different ways to express themselves, and themes are often linked to the time of year. For instance the summer term group in July might consider how to prepare for and manage the approaching school summer holidays. All staff and group members come back together for a plenary before sharing a meal together, and the evening ends at 9:30 pm. As with the children's days, activities vary, but the aim is to bring a group of young people together, some of whom know each other and some of whom are new, provide them with a positive group experience, and bring them back to a place where they can go home to their families.

Issues

The timing of the groups suits the young people, but is more difficult for their parents or carers. A 6:30 pm start is impossible for many working parents, and those who are caring for other younger children in the evening. This has prevented us from holding a concurrent parents group, and increased our reliance on the transport provided through St Christopher's. Volunteer drivers usually bring many of the young people in to the groups, and cabs are ordered to take them home at 9:30 pm. Without this service the group would be inaccessible to most of the young people. Young people who live outside our catchment area are unlikely to attend as the practicalities of the journey across London in the rush hour are too difficult.

There is a tension between the requirements for group safety and cohesion and stimulation in an on-going open group. Every group is different, as the attendance is always different, and the group has to reconstitute itself for every meeting. New members have to be introduced and included and old members also have to feel their issues are attended to. Both groups must feel they have gained enough from the evening to convince them to return to the next meeting, which may be several months hence.

Addressing this requires careful planning by the staff team, and detailed recording of attendance, activities, and process for each group. Group members who may have done activities previously are put in a small group or pair with a young person they do not know, and are often asked to be a buddy for a new member and help them with the exercise or activity. One young man on his first attendance following the death of his grandfather, was visibly moved by the story told by another member whose father had died, and asked her very directly but with great sensitivity how she had coped.

Another issue for an on-going group is when and how to negotiate members leaving. Although this is usually initiated by the young person when they feel they are ready and occurs without a formal goodbye, as is to be expected with a group that meets only three times a year, there are occasions when the group leaders have to make it happen.

Although some young people who attend the group seem to develop an accelerated maturity and understanding through their experience of the process of bereavement, for others the process of reconstitution takes them back to where they were developmentally before the bereavement (Christ 2000). These young people need to work through the adolescent tasks (Erikson 1963) which may have been put on hold while they focused on their grief, and they need to do this work outside the boundaries of a bereavement group.

In one example, a young man who had been attending for some time had explored his feelings about the death and resolved many of the issues it had raised for him, and was now more concerned with immediate issues at school and home. In the group he refused to engage in any of the activities and sabotaged the process for his small group. Any on-going group has to deal with the tension between holding on and letting go of members, and structures are needed to help both staff and members manage the transition. This situation had not risen before in the group's short history, and we now offer young people in this situation the following three options; they can simply stop attending, which happens in the majority of cases, they can have an informal leaving meeting with a Candle team member with a goodbye in a group meeting if they wish and the timing is right, or they can become more involved with facilitating and helping with the group, taking on more responsibilities for newer members and receiving support from staff in that role. If this last option proves successful we aim to work towards establishing a separate group of young volunteers, who could take part in all of our group events.

Parent/carer's childcare

The parent carers group is described in another chapter, and the child care provision has been one of the reasons for its continued popularity with members. Candle volunteers, supervised and co-ordinated by one of the team members, organize and plan the activities to occupy up to as many as 22 children for a two hour period on a Saturday while the group is taking place in a separate part of the building. These groups were established on a once a term basis, as the resources of the project could not stretch to more than three sessions per year, although the adults have often met at other times without child care.

Children as young as one and as old as fifteen have attended, but most are between six and 12 years. Children are able to try a variety of craft-based activities with the aim of producing something they can take home at the end of the session, most of which are the inspiration of one volunteer who has specific training and expertise in that field. If the weather permits there is also a trip to the park to play football, or some other energetic activity for those who do not want to do crafts.

Issues

Many of the children know each other quite well as they have been coming for several years, but the time between sessions can be as much as five months, which is a long time in the life of a young child, so their relationships remain at the level of acquaintance rather than close friendship.

The children display a sensitivity to each other's feelings that is perhaps unusual in such a disparate mix of age, class, education, race, and gender, and are able to learn strategies to cope with difficult situations that will arise for them within a safe environment. In one group, a cake had been produced for a child whose birthday was on that day. Another child, whose dead mother's birthday was also on the same day, had been asked when she arrived what she wanted to do about the celebrations. She thought for a moment and asked to sit on the outside of the group with a team member while the candles were lit and song was sung, but remain in the same room so that she could still be with the other children.

The sessions provide a very different experience for the volunteers to the more structured and intense children's days, and they appreciate the chance to build relationships with the children over time. The team member coordinates the volunteers, organizes the practicalities of venue, refreshments, and transport and is the responsible person in the case of emergency. She is able to leave the management of the session itself to the volunteers, and meets with them afterwards to debrief them.

Volunteers

The Candle project is part of St Christophers Hospice, and like the hospice, could not operate without volunteers. Volunteer drivers from the transport department bring children and families in to individual sessions and groups, and the Candle volunteer group are involved in all the groups we run. Selection, training, supervision, and support for volunteers is labour intensive (see Chapter 10). All the volunteers at Candle have been specifically recruited and Criminal Record Bureau checked and have received a 25 hour training programme on working with bereaved children in groups before they start, and on-going supervision and training while they remain part of the project. The staff team share this responsibility, and the sessional worker in the team specializes in working with the volunteers. This involves a lot of behind the scenes support by phone to remind and encourage busy and sometimes forgetful volunteers to commit themselves to the group days. We have always attempted to recruit volunteers who are as representative as possible of the local community. After their first interview, all the training, pre-group preparations, group activities, and supervision for volunteers take place outside of standard working hours at weekends or in the evenings, to enable people who work full time or have daytime commitments to apply. The volunteer group currently consists mainly of people with a professional background of some description, but within that a wide variety of different trainings, from law enforcement, teaching, childcare, and nursing to administration and physiotherapy. The volunteer group bring a richness and diversity of experience to the work, and children who attend the groups can experience support in bereavement delivered by people other than professional counsellors and therapists.

Supervision

Following the Saturday children's days there is a compulsory supervision session with the staff a few days later, which provides volunteers and staff a chance to explore in more depth some of the issues that may come up from the day. We are asking people to give up their evening, so for all the meetings with the volunteers we provide refreshments and allow some time for them to socialize as well. The staff team meet again separately for their supervision session following the meeting with the volunteers. The structure and expectations for supervision are the same for the specialist day groups for children bereaved by suicide and the workshop for parents and younger children.

For other groups that we run, for example the young people's evenings and the child-care sessions for the parent/carer groups, we hold short debriefing sessions immediately after the group members have left. This is for practical reasons, and in response to requests from volunteers, who were reluctant to give up another evening to attend supervision for a shorter group session.

The structure of the groupwork provision at Candle has developed in response to resource availability and client need. As I write this chapter I am aware of changes we have made and new groups we are currently planning. A system of one-off groups allows us to provide a swift and flexible response to the needs of families as they present and our resources allow. Candle has a small staff team, which makes communication easier and enables us to respond quickly to the changing needs for groupwork provision, and rooms are readily available within the hospice premises. Staff supervision sessions and monthly team meetings provide opportunities to review groupwork provision and plan new activities and events.

Families we see at Candle seem to appreciate the variety of provision and the different options available to them. Theoretically, a family with one teenaged and one younger child could be offered a choice from the bereaved parent/carer group, the young people's evening, the children's day, and the on-going parent/carer group as well as the individual and family support. The fact is that groups are offered but families are allowed to opt out, and the open one-off structure allows them to opt in again if and when they wish to. The groupwork demands on staff time are quite extensive, but fluctuating, allowing staff time in between activities to recover and reflect. Staff also appreciate the variety that the groupwork programme brings and the opportunity it offers to work with families in different ways. Volunteers bring fresh insights, skills, and energy to the team. The challenge of the groupwork programme is to remain flexible and inclusive, and to provide sufficient checks and balances within the basic structure to ensure that the experience is beneficial to all the children and families we work with.

References

Baulkwill J, Wood C (1995). In: S Smith, M Pennells (ed.) *Interventions with bereaved children.* London: Jessica Kingsley.

Childhood Bereavement Network (2002). *A death in the lives of ...* Nottingham: The Childhood Bereavement Network (VHS Video).

Childhood Bereavement Network, Mapping Exercise 2002.

Christ GH (2000). *Healing children's grief.* New York: Oxford University Press.

Dwivedi KN (ed.) (1993). *Group work with children and adolescents.* London: Jessica Kingsley.

Erikson E (1963). *Childhood and society.* London: Vintage.

Kane B (1979). Children's concepts of death. *Journal of Genetic Psychology* **134**:141–53.

Kirk K, McManus M (2002). Containing families' grief: therapeutic group work in a hospice setting. *International Journal of Palliative Nursing, 2002* **8**(10):470–80.

Lansdown R, Benjamin G (1985). The development of the concept of death in children aged 5-9 years. *Child Care, Health and Development* **11**:13–20.

Lloyd-Williams M, Wilkinson C, Lloyd-Williams F (1998). Do bereaved children consult the primary health care team more frequently? *European Journal of Cancer Care* **7**:120–24.

Lohnes Kelly L, Kalter N (1994). Preventative intervention groups for parentally bereaved children. *American Journal Orthopsychiatry* **64**(4):594–603.

Pfeffer CR, Jiang HR, Kakuma T *et al.* (2002). Group intervention for children bereaved by the suicide of a relative. *Journal of American Academy of Child Psychiatry, May 2002* **41**(5):505–13.

Smith SC, Pennells M (1995). *Interventions with bereaved children.* London: Jessica Kingsley.

Stokes J (2004). *Then now and always: supporting children as they journey through grief-a practitioner's guide.* Cheltenham: Winston's Wish.

Thompson F, Payne S (2000). Bereaved children's questions to a doctor. *Mortality* **5**(1):74–96.

Webb NB (ed.) (1993). *Helping Bereaved Children.* New York: Guilford Press.

Yalom I (1975). *Theory and Practice of Group Psychotherapy.* New York: Basic Books.

Chapter 7

Shrinking the space between people

Di Stubbs

The cornerstone of child bereavement work will always lie in the face-to-face and person-to-person connection that is made between practitioner and child or young person. Even though bereavement services for children and young people and their families have grown rapidly in the last ten years, we are a long way from the desired situation of every bereaved family having a truly local, open access service on their doorstep. And even if we do, one day, reach that Eden, there will always be families for whom individual or group work is not possible or appropriate.

However, almost everyone has access to a telephone, an increasing number of people have access to e-mail and the internet and many people use text messaging. Creative use of this technology can shrink the space between the practitioner and the bereaved person.

Early intervention

Telephone and e-mail support offer a new twist on the concept of early intervention in bereavement and trauma support. It is more traditional to see early intervention as a face-to-face interaction between the bereaved person and the practitioner, arranged soon after the death. However, where this is impossible for geographic or other logistical reasons, technology is making information, guidance, and support available. At the end of the line, at a click of a mouse, there can be a highly skilled and experienced practitioner who can make a timely, significant and lasting difference to bereaved families.

Leo called, concerned about his 12-year-old son, Kip, who had showed no emotion after his mother's death from breast cancer four months earlier. The practitioner explored how Leo was responding himself to his wife's death. Leo explained that he tried to keep things 'bouncing along', didn't mention his wife for fear of upsetting his son, kept his feelings under strict control until Kip was in bed and then cried into the night. The answerer gently asked how Kip might interpret his dad's reactions ... this 'hero' dad. There was an audible moment of realization. Leo immediately understood how his responses were telling Kip that men don't cry, don't mention people who die, and go on as usual. As he said 'how can he dare to cry if I'm always bright? How can he talk about her if I never do? Hey, I'm going to cry <u>with</u> him tonight.' 15 minutes had, hopefully, changed that family's communication and encouraged the therapeutic sharing of their individual griefs.

At the end of the line ...

The concept of helplines is over 50 years old but it has only been in comparatively recent years that the general public has thought of using the telephone to reach out for information, advice, guidance and, especially, emotional support. The phone offers several advantages over face-to-face encounters to a person seeking help for bereaved children–and themselves.

It would help to consider briefly, some characteristics of face-to-face work from the perspective of the bereaved person:

- usually an appointment system
- sometimes with a considerable waiting list
- within time-restrained hours (e.g. 9 am to 5 pm)
- either at your home or the office of the organization or some other 'clinical' space
- not available in some areas of the UK
- at least basic details about you and your family are known to the organization
- temptation to 'put on a brave face'
- you are likely to be affected by the other person's responses and reactions

For a bereaved person, exhausted both physically and emotionally, it can be an enormous effort to take the necessary actions to arrive at a face-to-face meeting. There is the concern that you may be judged by your appearance (age, weight, gender, ethnic background, physical ability, health, etc). You may feel that you should ask how the practitioner is feeling and that may prevent you from saying something that might upset the kind stranger in front of you.

Advantages of telephone support–for the person making contact

- control—feeling you are in control of the communication; you can even ring off before speaking
- anonymity—you do not have to give a name or a location
- immediacy—you can call when you want or need to, subject to the helpline's opening hours, no need to make an appointment
- accessibility—you can make contact from anywhere with a phone or almost anywhere with a mobile

- ease of contact—you don't have to tidy the living room or even get dressed to make contact
- emotion—if you are uncomfortable with expressing emotion, it may be easier to talk without being face-to-face with someone
- one-way—you are the focus of the call, you don't have to consider how the other person is reacting to what you say
- endings—you can ring off at any time with no embarrassment or apology.

Disadvantages–for the person making contact

- no visual clues on the response coming from the other person—e.g. shock, sympathy
- some people find it harder to communicate and harder to decide whether to trust without seeing the other person

Advantages—for the person answering

- focus on what is being said (and not said) without visual distractions
- easier to ask the more difficult questions or explore the more painful areas
- nature of the contact (spontaneity and intimacy) can lead to a more quickly established rapport
- location—the answerer does not need to leave the office
- the answerer can make notes, look out of the window or sip a cup of tea without appearing impolite or uninterested

Disadvantages—for the person answering

- no visual clues that can guide response—are they silently struggling?
- accents can be harder to decipher over the phone

An intimate disclosure

Some people think that it must feel impersonal talking to a helpline; in practice, most callers find a special intimacy in talking over the phone to someone who makes the time to listen and is felt to care. A caller once described it as 'whispering your pain into someone's ear'. Of course, the quality of the intervention—over the phone as much as in a face-to-face encounter—is determined by the way in which the answerer (or practitioner) is able to create for the caller a place that feels safe for the sharing of powerful feelings.

The caller ('you') has overcome the first barrier to seeking support and guidance by picking up the phone and dialing the number. While this can be incredibly hard to do—at least it allows you the chance to ring off, to keep silent for a while, to decide whether you trust the tone of this voice. In a phone communication, tone is what matters most. The right tone transcends accent, class, gender. The right-toned voice can make you stay and talk when you were poised to ring off.

If the voice at the end of the line sounds warm without seeming cloying, unhurried without seeming un-bothered, accepting without seeming uncaring, and concerned without seeming intrusive then you are more likely to trust it with your deepest feelings. If the voice is also able to convey a kindly, informed competence and a trustworthy reliability, the relationship between caller and called stands a chance. Most of all, does this voice 'stand alongside' you in your pain and confusion and sound as if it will support your choices and actions?

When Chad Varah, the Founder of the Samaritans, was first selecting volunteers to befriend over the phone, he asked himself 'Could I tell this voice the most awful, oppressive, dark secret of my life?' A 'yes' usually ensured acceptance.

So, the right voice—or the right-enough voice—answers; what then? This will depend a little on who you are. In seeking support for a bereaved child or young person, you may be in one (or more) of these groups:

◆ parent, carer, or guardian

◆ other relative, family friend, or neighbour

◆ teacher or tutor

◆ concerned professional

   ◆ health care

   ◆ social care

   ◆ coroner; funeral director, etc.

   ◆ police Family Liaison Officer

   ◆ faith leader

◆ a child or young person.

For the sake of exploring the helpline intervention further, I am going to assume that the caller is a parent or key carer of a child whose parent or sibling has died.

What happens next may depend on the type of helpline you have contacted and how it is staffed. Helplines may be answered by trained practitioners or by trained volunteers. These volunteers may or may not have experienced bereavement themselves. Helplines may solely offer advice and information or signposting to other sources of support. Others may focus on providing emotional support.

All of these have been tried within the wider field of bereavement support and all have their place. What will vary will be the degree to which the guidance and information is based on practice as well as theory, the access to linked services and resources and also whether the sharing of personal information by the answerer is considered appropriate. In practice, when providing bereavement support to an adult supporting a bereaved child, a conversation will range over many areas. It may start by listening, emotional support, and befriending, move through some information about children and grief, offer some guidance or direct advice, and end with some practical ideas and some more emotional support.

Outcomes

In offering bereavement support over the phone, it is good to consider what the outcome of a call may be for the caller. This can then become a measurement by which to evaluate how the call went. A reasonable outcome might be that the concerned adult feels better able, after the call, to support the bereaved child. This, in turn, would mean that the bereaved child or young person is better able to journey through their grief.

To break this down further, it may be that, after the call, the family will be better able to communicate and to express their thoughts and feelings of grief. They will also feel encouraged to preserve memories of the person who has died. In addition, the call may give the caller a widened understanding of death in general and this death in particular and a wider appreciation of the needs and responses of bereaved children.

Answering the call

It is important for those answering the call to remember (for the caller we are assuming the parent or carer of a bereaved child) that this is, therefore, someone who is experiencing their own bereavement. The child may have lost a parent, a sibling, a grandparent. The caller will have lost a partner, an ex-partner, a child, a parent.

> When his Grandfather died, my son said solemnly 'I'm a bereaved child' and I thought 'so am I' (caller to helpline)

Recognizing that a key element of how a child or young person will respond to the death of someone important is the response of the parent or key carer, in any intervention we need to have a concern for the person in the parental role. Support for them will help secure a better outcome for their family.

After the caller has decided to trust this voice, the task of relationship is not over. It has to be continually remade throughout the call. This requires a very active form of listening; the answerer must sit up and listen, not sit back and listen. The quality of the listening elicits what the caller wants to say. A helpline answerer has highly privileged access to the caller's thoughts and feelings and has to use this access with great care and consideration.

All good helpline answerers use similar equipment and tools. For example:

- the use of open-ended questions
- reflecting back what the caller has said
- summarizing
- asking what they had thought of doing or saying
- the creative use of 'mmmm' and 'mmm?'
- 'don't just do something, sit there'
- the therapeutic use of silence.

So your pain has been heard and the answerer has begun gently to focus on the children and young people who have been bereaved. At this point in a helpline call with a bereaved family, the practitioner is conducting an assessment. This may be a partial one, a one-sided one, or a brief one—but it is nevertheless an assessment along remarkably similar lines to that outlined in Chapter 3.

In brief, the answerer is assessing what this death means to this child or children, at this time, living in this family and in this community.

Most of this information is usually offered by the caller without prompting and occurs spontaneously within the conversation.

The next question the answerer needs to ask themselves is 'what help/support/guidance is this family asking me for?'. The subsequent question is 'what do I think this family needs?'. It can be quite a temptation to put these two questions the other way around but it is important to respect and honour the caller's autonomy and put their needs first.

This may now be the time to offer some information, for example, about children's differing developmental understanding of death, about common reactions and responses, about the thoughts and feelings of grief. And after the sharing of information, comes the time for advice or guidance. The intention needs to be to offer any guidance tentatively, always being aware that bereaved people attract well-meaning but infuriating advice as a honey pot attracts bees. The helpline answerer will avoid saying 'if I were you …' or 'why don't you? … or 'what you need to do now is …' Instead they will try some of these approaches. 'What have you thought of doing …?' 'You may want to consider …' 'Some people find it helps to …' 'I wonder if you'd thought of …' 'What would happen if you …' 'How do you think your child would react if you …' The answerer must always keep in mind that this family is operating and needs to operate within their own family context—past, present, and future.

The next stage of the helpline call can then be offering practical ideas. These are powerful, creative tools and resources to help the family at this time. These include suggesting activities such as making a memory box or book and offering ideas for ways to remember someone who has died at Christmas/Father's Day/their birthday etc. This is also the time when other resources can be suggested; books or other printed materials, useful websites, child bereavement services in the caller's locality, or—if local to the helpline and appropriate to the caller—the time to explore how the service may be able to offer one to one or group support.

The approaching end of the call gives the answerer a chance to summarize, to reflect back, to remind of any key points or actions, and a chance to check that the caller has said all they want to. It is also the time to encourage the caller to call again, if this is appropriate; to acknowledge their grief and sense of loss; to pay tribute to their care and concern for the children amidst their own grief, and to convey the telephonic equivalent of a warm hand clasp.

At the end of the call, the answerer needs to reflect on what has been shared and learned, take any necessary actions (for example, sending resources), follow agreed practices on recording the call and, importantly, seek any support they need for themselves.

Some calls demand every ounce of the answerer's attention, skill, knowledge, and empathy. It is essential that the organization has a support mechanism in place for the 'coming down' phase, if required. 'Debriefing' will involve allowing the answerer to describe the call, the family's situation, what was discussed, and any actions that need to be taken. Equally important is the chance to describe their personal responses and to consider how they feel they were able to support the caller. Immediately after a difficult call is the time for encouragement, and also for straightforward acknowledgement of the answerer's feelings. Further opportunity to discuss the calls should always be on offer – either within regular supervision or as an informal offer from other staff.

It must not be assumed that a helpline can meet every caller's needs. A final point concerns the times when things go less smoothly. These are some of those possibilities:

◆ Callers who misunderstand the nature of the helpline service and wish it to provide something else, for example a free holiday

◆ Callers whose demands on the service are greater than can be met, for example those who wish to ring several times a day

◆ Callers who express serious suicidal intent

◆ Callers who intend to harm their children or other people; or when reference is made to physical, sexual, or emotional abuse.

◆ Callers who appear to seek to disrupt the HelpLine.

All organizations that provide helplines have to establish policies that will address these issues, and need to provide training for helpline answerers. Confidentiality and child protection procedures have to be considered within the helpline context. Skills practice (role play) is useful for those learning how to deal with the demanding caller and how to set out the limits of the service clearly and unambiguously without alienating the caller.

Calls from children and young people

Although having written mainly about receiving calls from adults, it is important to consider calls from young people. Helplines may actively seek calls from bereaved young people (for example, within the UK, lines operated by Cruse and by ChildLine) or, at the least, need to anticipate receiving and responding to them.

Particular training is necessary when preparing to receive calls from children and young people. While, in theory, there may be little or no difference between supporting children or adults who are grieving; in reality, a phone answerer may find themselves becoming involved and affected more quickly and more deeply when talking by phone to a child who is grieving. The use of skills practice (role play) is again very valuable. Discussion is vital on potential situations that may, or will challenge policies and procedures. For example, what if a young caller talks about their drug use or suicide attempts? What if they tell of a bereaved sibling being physically abused? What if they have deliberately not told their name or address but have let slip the name of their school?

When supporting children over the phone, it is important to be realistic and honest with ourselves as well as with them about the limits of what we can do. The telephone offers a tremendous opportunity to engage young people who may feel more confident at speaking to someone they can't see. It also offers a good opportunity to give support at a distance over a longer period by regular, possibly short, contacts between the bereaved young person and the practitioner who is working with them. No need to come out of classes, no problem with a sudden after school activity—just a catch-up, 'how are you?' call at a convenient time.

The Winston's Wish Family Line (0845 2030405)

The question of how to reach more families with an early intervention is what prompted Winston's Wish (a community-based child bereavement organization) to launch a national helpline in the UK for anyone caring for a bereaved child. By the end of the first three years (March 2001–February 2004), over 12 500 people had contacted the service by phone. These people, in turn, were concerned about around 25 000 bereaved children and young people. In the same three-year period (March 2001–February 2004), we met around 750 bereaved children and their families and around 420 children and 180 adults were involved in 18 residential weekends.

It is obviously fairly meaningless to compare the two interventions solely in terms of numbers. However, our experience shows that assumptions about the difference in depth, quality, and impact of the intervention may not be valid. Thirty minutes' phone conversation with a trained and experienced child bereavement practitioner may revolutionize a person's response to their child and that child's needs.

We decided that our own staff would answer the Winston's Wish Family Line: this ensures that every call from any type of caller is answered by an experienced practitioner. That is, the calls are answered by the same person who, later in the day, will get down on the floor to draw with a 6-year-old, the same person who will co-ordinate Camp Winston, the same person who can go alongside an angry adolescent or despairing parent or guardian. This, we believe, adds quality to the intervention and the combination of both a theoretical and experiential basis gives us the ability to offer a wide-reaching and comprehensive service.

The helpline is aimed at supporting adults and our publicity carries the line: 'Are you caring for a bereaved child?' This allows potential callers to define our primary audience for themselves in terms of their relationship to the child under concern and the child's relationship to the person who has died.

We receive more calls from family members than any other group (77% from the family: 23% from professionals). Of family callers, more mothers call than fathers, with grandparents and step relations being the next largest groups of family members. Twenty-six familial relationships have been described by callers, for example great aunt, second cousin and 'ex-step-grandmother'. Professional callers include health and social care professionals, teachers and educational workers, police family liaison officers, faith leaders, and counsellors.

More details on this helpline can be found in 'Then, Now and Always' Stokes JA, 2004, Winston's Wish Publication.

At the click of a mouse...

In 1993, Steve Harris, a Samaritans volunteer in Cheltenham, England, began to imagine how the Samaritans' emotional support could be offered through e-mail. It is a little humbling to have to acknowledge that when he and his Branch Director brought the idea of an e-mail befriending scheme to the General Office, it was this author who, at that time, felt there was 'no future' in the idea! Happily, they persisted and persuaded, and the e-mail befriending scheme was launched in 1994. E-mail befriending is the fastest growing area of Samaritans contacts with around 80 000 e-mails received in 2002.

Many organizations now actively offer support, guidance, and information through e-mail; and others are contacted by e-mail. For organizations and groups seeking to support bereaved children, young people and their families, the provision of support through e-mail has to be at least considered since it will be the contact method of choice of much of their target audience.

There are advantages and disadvantages of communicating through e-mail both for the person making contact and for the therapeutic answerer.

Advantages—for the person making contact

- Control—over content and over ending contact
- Anonymity
- Immediacy and speed
- Accessibility—you can e-mail and access replies from anywhere with an internet connection and e-mail is increasingly used by those with speech and/or hearing difficulties
- Privacy
- One way (when you want a response but do not want a conversation)
- Cost advantage
- Normality—most young people and an increasing percentage of the population use e-mail as the communication medium of choice
- Written word—it can be easier emotionally and less embarrassing to write rather than to say, you can review what you've written before sending it.

Disadvantages—for person making contact

- No clues on the response coming from the other person—shock, sympathy
- Have to wait for response when the emotional need may be urgent
- Some people find it harder to put thoughts and feelings into words on paper

Advantages—for the person answering

- Content—all the content of the communication is available from the outset
- Feelings and thoughts—'you get deeper quicker'; strong emotions do not feel personal on the page
- Quality—the response can be improved by checking over each word and, if required, checking response with someone else before sending it
- Voices—no struggling with quiet voices, regional accents, etc.
- Less judgemental—response not clouded by judgements made on clues in the caller's voice
- Environment—you are not distracted by surrounding noise as with phone calls
- Location and timing—you can respond from anywhere with a net connection and you can, within reason, choose when to reply
- Priority—you can prioritize responses to several e-mails
- Re-contact—you have the enquirer's address so can follow-up, sensitively, if there is no reply

Disadvantages—for answerer

- Lack of clues—to guide responses, lack of cultural reference points, lack of nuance can make it harder to grasp what is being said
- Urgency—harder to assess the urgency of the need
- Spontaneity—the delay between contact and response cuts the potential for a spontaneous reaction; it also takes time for answers to any questions to arrive
- Warmth—harder to convey warmth and empathy through the written word
- Silence–it isn't possible to 'use' silence
- Mistakes—harder to pull the conversation round if you make a mistake/misinterpretation and also having a written record of your response may lead to over caution

To e or not to e

There are important considerations for a service that intends to communicate with bereaved people by e-mail. In outlining some of these, I will be referring to our experience at Winston's Wish. Within our service to bereaved families, we receive e-mails from bereaved young people as well as from their parents, carers, or other family members, and from professionals. The majority come through our website within which there are several opportunities to ask a question; however a significant proportion come directly to the organization.

Who will be e-mailing you ?

It is important to be clear about who your primary 'audience' for support is <u>intended</u> to be so that you can plan the service to meet their needs. However, in practice, whoever it is aimed at, you will receive e-mails from people in other groups (parents, young people, professionals) as well as from the researcher, journalist, and the person who has 'come to the wrong shop'. The following points will concentrate mainly on responding to e-mails from young people.

Who will respond ?

Because e-mail is so much part of our world, it may be thought that there is no need for special training in replying. However, it takes real skill and experience to be able to make an assessment of the e-mail writer's needs and feelings—both the stated and unstated–and to respond supportively. Additional training in using the written word therapeutically is required; also the medium itself allows the possibility of consultation on a response that is not possible with a phone call or face-to-face work.

It might be assumed that e-mail support is best handled by younger people. In practice, older people may even be more comfortable and familiar with responding using the written word (i.e. writing a letter) so assumptions should not be made.

Responding to e-mails is an integral part of the service being provided to bereaved young people—not an 'add-on'. It can be handled by someone at a remote location. For example, in the experience of the Samaritans, a person who e-mails their despair to jo@samaritans.org.uk, will receive a reply within 24 hours from one of 118 branches, throughout the world. An e-mailer from Huddersfield may be answered in Hong Kong.

E-mail responding probably works best when handled by the whole team as a standard part of their work, recognizing that this carries training implications (including in the use of computers). For organizations expecting a large volume of calls, software is now available to route received e-mails to answerers in several locations.

Having a generic e-mail address for young people to contact such as 'info@xxx' or 'ask@xxx' can help the feeling that it is the whole organization that cares and is offering support rather than one individual. This same address can then be used for replies. It is then important to decide how each e-mail will be signed. I would recommend a standard name for use by all – at Winston's Wish, all e-mails are answered by 'Chris'.

If we were to describe how we would like those who e-mail us to think of the person who responds to e-mails at Winston's Wish, we would hope they would characterize them as something like an ideal big brother or favourite aunt who can be supportive of all thoughts and feelings, caring without being suffocating, has helpful information but is not going to lecture, knows a bit more about the world than you but is not going to preach about it, and is fundamentally on your side.

When will they respond?

It is also important to have an agreed response time (we currently promise a reply within 24 hours of receiving the e-mail question). It is possible to generate an automatic response so that the sender knows that their question has been received and approximately when they can expect an answer.

Policies, practices, and procedures

E-mail response should be an integral part of any service, subject to the same policies, practices, and procedures as face to face or group work. In addition to those mentioned before, these need to include a policy on data protection, record keeping, and storage.

Policies may need to be re-considered in the light of e-mail support. Here are some questions to consider:

◆ How can you enact your child protection policy if you do not know the child's location?

◆ How do you support a suicidal young person when you do not know their location?

◆ To what extent are you prepared to use security or other systems to trace someone?

◆ How mindful do you need to be in your response of the possibility of someone else reading it?

◆ If you are offering advice that can be printed out and kept, do you need to have indemnity insurance?

◆ For how long will you keep records? And will you keep these electronically or on paper?

◆ How do you ensure continuity if your service starts an e-mail 'conversation' with someone (i.e. they reply to your reply…)?

◆ What are the boundaries of subjects/issues you can and can not deal with by e-mail? How can you explain this to those who contact you?

◆ Will you include weblinks to useful websites? How will you decide what is suitable and/or useful?

What makes e-mail support particularly appropriate for young people who have been bereaved?

We know, while acknowledging the generalization, that young people can find it hard to seek support from a stranger face-to-face. Even those close to them may struggle to reach a point of easy communication about thoughts and feelings of grief. Yet, every day, it is estimated (2004) that around 25 billion e-mails are sent around the world—a sizeable proportion of these are sent by young people to each other. There is something about the process that has an attractive ambivalence–using the hardware to express something softer. The communication takes place at a distance through tapping on a keyboard—yet it feels like an intimate connection. It has all the advantages outlined above, immediate, convenient, tentative, fleeting—that makes it suit a young person who is unsure about seeking support following bereavement.

Recognizing the language

E-mail is increasingly used by young people to communicate and is developing a language of its own that is linked to text messaging. It is a vibrant, direct, and immediate language that is suited to the communication of feelings and thoughts. It is unlikely that an e-mail message will be correctly spelt or grammatical but it will be powerful. For example:

> My dad died nearly a yer ago .And scince then my life feel rubish .and i somtimes just want to die. When will i stop like this?

> it is my mum who has died she died of a brain hemeridge it was all sudden. i live with my dad i have no brothers or sisters i am 12 years off age my bday is today

In replying to an e-mail from a young person, it is not necessary to use the same language – for example, to deliberately mis-spell a word to seem 'cool' and 'in touch'; but it is necessary to be direct, non-fussy and non-academic. It would probably help, however, to have some grasp of commonly used acronyms, shorthand, and emoticons. If in doubt, ask a teenager to help!

It would also aid consistency to have available some standard paragraphs (for example, how you describe your service) to go within the individual response and to use a standard font colour and size.

Parents and professionals

E-mails will also be received from adults seeking help for bereaved children. The same considerations apply to replies; it may also be the opportunity to direct them to telephone helplines and/or to local services.

The future for e-mail

E-mail support will become an important part of any child bereavement service within the next five years. Through e-mail we can reach bereaved young people whom we may struggle to reach in more traditional ways and offer them a warm, human response to their grief.

Using the worldwide web to reach young people

One of the real challenges for a child bereavement service is to engage children, young people, and their parents by finding a variety of communications that will work for all ages. Within the last few years, there has been an incredible shift in how we access information, support, and even company. For those with access to the Internet (100% of young people–if you include access at school and/or library), it is now usually the first choice for those seeking to understand more about a subject or seek support.

A website is, nowadays, a necessary requirement for any organization seeking to have any public profile. But it can also become so much more than simply a promotion of the organization's existence.

Aims

When we designed the website for Winston's Wish, we wanted to achieve four distinct things. For us, the first and strongest reason to have a website is as a means of engaging bereaved young people in the 11–18 age range. We had become aware that, despite creative measures, this group was less likely to participate in one-to-one work and in group work than their younger counterparts. Secondly, we wanted to put information and guidance on supporting bereaved children and young people into the public domain where parents and carers, professionals and schools could instantly access it. Thirdly, we wanted to increase our public profile and fourthly, we hoped to expand fund-raising support through e-commerce.

The youth pages of any website need to develop as an integral part of the services on offer and need to contribute to realizing the vision that all bereaved children receive the support they need to manage the impact of death in their lives. Additionally, they may also provide an insight into young people's responses and reactions to a wider audience, for example their parent(s), professionals, and students.

There is, of course, no control that says only young people will access pages aimed at young people; equally you can assume that young people will explore throughout the site and need to feel acknowledged and respected wherever they go.

Why a website?

Web pages have many potential advantages for bereaved young people providing:

- anonymity—nobody knowing who is accessing the pages
- privacy—nobody looking over your shoulder at your emotions
- ease of access—no appointment system or library check-out to negotiate
- immediacy—there at the click of a mouse
- accessibility—accessible to all regardless of physical ability, race, culture, gender
- availability—available 24-7
- one-to-machine—no obvious contact with another person

- freedom of expression—no need to feel bad if you rush off somewhere else or swear vehemently

- culturally relevant—meeting young people on their own 'ground'.

Searching for help

A website can become one of the first opportunities to reach the bereaved. The enquirer may be looking specifically for immediate information about our particular service by name and known web address, maybe prior to contacting us directly or instead of doing so. Alternatively, the enquirer may tap key words such as 'bereavement' 'grief' 'death' 'children' into a search engine and find a service that way.

The young person's perspective

You can imagine a bereaved teenager, sitting at the computer in their room or even at school. Feeling very diffident, very suspicious, very reluctant. Looking at the screen and then steeling themselves to either search for information in general or to look specifically at a known child bereavement service site. They will be poised to leave at every second as the site loads; their antennae will be alert for signs of patronizing, preaching, or 'poor-little-you' sympathy.

We have to be aware that it is incredibly quick and easy to click away from a website about bereavement and onto something more enticing. We have to design sites that will convey rapidly the ethos of our service to reassure and encourage young people who are internet-literate and critical. And then we have to meet at least some of the needs that young people will bring to the site.

Young bereaved people will probably expect a website about bereavement services to talk down to them and tell them what to do, to be falsely comforting, to be over-cheery or over-serious, to be boring and worthy. Therefore the tone of any website or youth pages within an organization's website need to convey the qualities of the service, for example, that this service is approachable, trustworthy, and accepting of people's feelings and thoughts.

Using computers is, of course, not appropriate for all young people. Also, pages aimed at young people–like all good website content–need to be accessible to those with impaired sight or hearing and to young people with low literacy levels or for whom English is not their first language.

Logging out

The website may seek to encourage a young person to return on another occasion by having features that are sufficiently helpful, or may change, or are interactive. When they click away from the site, it would be good if they felt that they had been accepted, respected, and supported.

Actually, I don't like to admit it, but I felt a bit better afterwards.

I talked to mum about dad for the first time since he died.

I'll have a look tomorrow to see if anyone else feels like me.

www.winstonswish.org.uk

Like most organizations, the Winston's Wish website provides a window to the range of services available. We strive to make the standard features of these 'corporate' pages clear and striking for interested parties and potential supporters. We have, however, developed a large interactive and moderated section within our website specifically aimed at young people.

Content

Through this area of the site, bereaved young people are able to engage in a variety of interactive activities around remembering the person who has died and expressing feelings and thoughts of grief. They can gain access to information about death, dying, and bereavement. Young people can also communicate with us by asking a specific question or with each other through moderated message boards.

It is almost impossible to describe a rapidly-developing website in words alone, so may I direct readers to the website (www.winstonswish.org.uk) for a longer look.

Other bereavement organizations are developing innovative content for young people. Worthy of particular mention is the site www.rd4u.org.uk, which is designed and updated by bereaved young people themselves.

The web has transformed our communication with each other but it is not a magic answer in itself. The development of a website does not remove the need to develop and deliver other direct services for bereaved teenagers.

HRU? RUOK? (How are you? Are you OK?)

Another possibility to add to our opportunities to reach bereaved people is the use of text messaging. Again, this is a technology that has almost universal acceptance amongst young people and is gradually being used by people of all ages.

When writing about responding to e-mails, I said that it was not necessary to use the same language in response. This is probably not true when it comes to text messaging and it would help to have a grasp of the acronyms and emoticons. If you don't have a convenient teenager on hand to translate, there are websites that can provide you with some commonly used expressions (IYKWIM! *If you know what I mean*).

Responding to text messages should be part of the overall package of services offered and, ideally, could be the role of all staff and volunteers. There needs to be training, adapted policies, procedures, consistency, quality control, monitoring, etc. The text above relating to responding to e-mails is relevant here. Texting has the advantages of e-mail to young people (please see previous list on page 105).

Most charities that have explored the use of text messaging have been looking at the potential for fund-raising or to create a community of supporters. Here are some first thoughts on how we could use text messaging to support bereaved young people. (FYI! *For your information.*)

With young people we already know

◆ A message on an important day—anniversary of the death, birthday of the person who has died, etc.

- A gentle 'thinking of you' message when you know they are going through a rough time
- An encouraging reminder of the next appointment or group meeting
- A follow-up to an individual session—'good to see you today'.

With young people new to our service

- A first point of contact for someone exploring the service. ('Text INFO to 07979 xxxx'.) The response could start a supportive connection for the young person.
- An opportunity to participate in a survey (e.g. of responses to bereavement), leading to a supportive connection.

Conclusion

It could be said that the provision of emotional support is at its purest between two people—one who needs support and one who cares to give it—irrespective of their ages, genders, nationalities, and even location. This chapter has looked at how we can use technology to provide relevant services to bereaved young people, their families, and the professionals who care for them.

For many adults, a helpline call, an e-mail or a read through a web page will be sufficient to enable them to continue to support their bereaved children. For some, the call, mail or page will point them to fresh ideas, new insights, and useful resources. For a few, the technology will act as a gateway to the services available nationally and locally. For young people, e-mails, texts, and websites may be the most bearable way to make the first tentative approach for help and support.

The technology is succeeding in shrinking the space between people.

Chapter 8

The extended warranty

Frances Kraus

The title of this book is intended to reflect the reality of work with bereaved children and families. Professionals and volunteers in the field are aware that for many bereaved families, a brief intervention will be the only one possible. The reasons are varied; for example, they can arise from the difficulties that bereaved families encounter in juggling the practical requirements of their everyday lives with their need to allow space and time to grieve, or from the limitations imposed by professional or volunteer bereavement workers who have to ration scarce resources. The Candle project followed the pattern of short-term intervention in bereavement that had worked well in a bereavement service already offered by St Christopher's Hospice. This service had confirmed our belief that, provided the service is delivered swiftly when requested, so that help is available when families are most receptive, short-term work is appropriate for the majority of bereaved children and families. Bereavement is a normal process of adjustment to a major life event, and attending counselling sessions long term can reduce a family's coping skills by creating a dependency on the bereavement counsellor or agency. Children form close relationships very quickly, and the ending of a long-term counselling relationship can give them another loss to cope with.

In common with many agencies in the bereavement field, Candle has engaged with the difficulties of providing a short-term intervention, while recognizing that for some families issues may arise in the future which require further help. In this chapter, I intend to look at the development of the idea of the extended warranty, a term I have borrowed from the insurance field, where it is used to mean an extension of the usual term of guarantee for a new purchase. The Candle extended warranty developed as a response to the problems and issues that can arise for bereaved families who have received a short-term intervention by offering the opportunity for further contact when needed.

Some families have problems that pre-date the bereavement, which make it impossible for them to focus on processing the grief, and these issues often become further complicated by the impact of the death on family life. Dora Black (2002), identifies children who are in the high risk groups following bereavement as follows:

- Children under 10 years
- Those with learning difficulties
- Those who have suffered previous losses

- Where there is a family or personal history of psychiatric disorder
- Where the death is sudden or otherwise traumatic
- Children who witness violent deaths of those known to them (homicide, accident, murder)
- Where there is a perceived threat to the child's own life
- Families where there are multiple adversities
- Families where the surviving parent[s] are failing in their care of the child.

Some or many of the above factors apply to a significant number of the children we see at Candle, and those with higher numbers of stressors need much more support than the short-term intervention the Candle project can provide. In this case, Candle staff assess the child and family and make a referral on to another agency such as the Child and Adolescent Mental Health Service, with the permission of the parent or carer.

The work of the Harvard Child Bereavement Study (Worden 1996), established that parental competence was a significant factor in determining a child's ability to cope with the experience of death. This finding was echoed in the later study of the effects of parental bereavement by Christ (2000). Christ followed 88 families through the terminal illness of the parent until 14 months after the death. Christ emphasized the importance of recognition of the 'cascade of events' that can happen after a bereavement, some of which may be more harmful to the child than the death itself. This term describes the secondary losses that occur for many children. Pre-existing problems in the child's life could be exacerbated by the bereavement, and the ability of the surviving parent to manage the child's grief as well as their own as well as all the other changes and adjustments was critical. Supporting parents as well as children has been central to the work of the Candle project.

The St Christopher's Candle project

The Candle project is an 'open access' service for bereaved children, based in St Christopher's Hospice in London. We accept referrals for children bereaved by death from any cause from families themselves, from professionals, and from volunteers. The geographical area we cover in South East London is a mixture of inner city boroughs with high levels of socio-economic deprivation and relatively affluent outer suburbs, with a very diverse cultural and ethnic mix. Overall, the proportion of children referred to Candle from all the black and minority ethnic communities is 35%, which reflects the ethnic mix across the area, bearing in mind that this is a project concerned with a young population. About 75% of the children referred to Candle are bereaved by a sudden or unexpected death, mostly through a sudden illness such as a heart attack, stroke, or brain haemorrhage, but also by a road traffic collision, suicide, or murder. The majority of the deaths (65%) are of a parent, but also include siblings, close relatives and care givers, and friends. Many of the families we work with are separated, which often complicates the process of bereavement, as the surviving parent or care giver may be unable to identify with and support their child's grief for a former partner. Many of our clients are coping with a stress factor such as poverty or mental illness before the death, and are less likely to be well supported following it. They come within the categories of children at risk in bereavement defined by Black (2002). This does not negate the value of a focused bereavement intervention in itself, but underlines the importance of the timing of the referral, the assessment process, and the capacity to refer on to other agencies.

Sometimes children are referred before a full assessment of their situation has been made. Families who have had negative experiences with statutory services are also more likely to approach a voluntary sector project directly, and Candle has a policy to encourage direct referrals from families. Many referrals come to Candle through schools, either directly from teachers or other school-based professionals such as school nurses or Special Educational Needs Co-ordinators, or indirectly by the school making the suggestion to the parent that they contact us. School staff often know less about the lives of their pupils outside school than might be supposed, and are sometimes unaware of other issues that may exist. Candle makes a number of referrals to the Child Trauma Stress Clinic, Social Services, or the Child and Adolescent Mental Health Services every year.

> A young man killed himself while in prison on remand for drug-related offences. He was felt by his family to be mentally ill at the time, and they demanded answers about what they felt was the lack of care he received in custody. His former partner, Sue, referred herself to the Candle project two months later with his two children, boys of 4 and 9 years old. She had experienced many difficulties while in the relationship with the children's father, eventually separating from him in order to stay away from the drug using culture. The death placed an intolerable burden upon her. Her partner's family blamed her for his death, which they attributed to his inability to cope with her leaving him. This meant that she lost much of her social support, and the children lost contact with some members of the family. Visits to some other family members were experienced by them as difficult due to the intensity of anger, blame, and recriminations they overheard. Sue was unable to cope with her older son's aggressive, demanding behaviour, which was also causing problems at school, and could not protect his younger brother, who was the target for much of the aggression. We did not feel that a short-term piece of bereavement work was appropriate at that time, as there were so many pre-existing and current issues, and made a referral to the Child and Adolescent Mental Health Service, who were able to offer support through several months of family therapy. The children returned to the project 18 months later and were given several sessions of bereavement work.

The case study illustrates the value of assessment, and of the ability to provide an appropriate referral to statutory agencies. We have found that maintaining a clear sense of our role, including our limitations, but at the same time making every attempt to assist families to get the help that they need has been much appreciated. We have learned never to underestimate the value of a well-considered report or assessment for a child in need of psychological help, and the accessibility of the service (most new referrals are contacted within two weeks), is in itself helpful to families under stress.

Fortunately, most of the children referred to the project are not trying to manage as many issues. There are, however, certain distinguishing factors about a child's grief that determined the way we developed the Candle extended warranty. The first is clearly based in child development. The comprehensive overview of the impact of bereavement on children at different stages of development in Christ's work (2000) emphasizes how a child's age and stage of development determine their reactions to bereavement and the ways adults around them can help. This is a dynamic process, and a child whose parent or close relative dies when they are six will need to revisit that loss as they grow physically, emotionally, and cognitively.

The other issue for children is their dependence on the adults around them. Children have little control over what happens to them, and need assistance to manage the effects of changes they may not have wished for or been consulted about. This is the case for all children, and part of growing up is learning how to adjust to new circumstances. Many adults, for example, can remember leaving primary school, where they were part of the oldest group of pupils, and moving to secondary school to become one of the youngest and newest. This experience of change is common for most adults in the United Kingdom, where primary and secondary schools are separate institutions, occupying different sites, and is remembered by some as exciting and liberating and by others as overwhelming. Changing school, and the emotional reactions that result, has to be managed by the child with the help of parents and carers, who will provide information, reassurance, and support. Bereaved children have to make these kinds of adjustments all the time, without the help of the person who has died.

The cascade of secondary losses, which is one of the compounding variables that makes evaluating bereavement interventions with children so hard (Stokes *et al.* 1997) provides many examples of issues a bereaved child will have to deal with; changes in responsibilities at home, changes in care givers, moving house or school, new step parents and siblings. These are often the reasons that prompt families to take up the offer of the extended warranty of Candle and return to the place that has been able to offer help initially and with whom they have a relationship of trust.

All of us like to think that we are important to the people with whom we come into contact and who offer us support at difficult times, and the knowledge that the project is there, 'holding in mind' the family or child's needs, can often serve as a confidence booster in itself. I still receive a Christmas card every year from a family I worked with nearly ten years ago as part of a short-term counselling service before the Candle project was in existence. The father had died in a road traffic crash, leaving a wife and two young children. The family have now moved to another part of the country, and although I have written back, Jean (the parent) does not reply, which suggests to me that her contact is a way of her telling herself as well as me that she is OK.

There are several issues to be considered when an extended warranty is offered. I will address these in the rest of this chapter, and illustrate with examples.

How to use the short-term context to encourage independence?

Bereaved families are vulnerable. An agency that is there for them, understanding their needs, and appreciating their problems and limitations is a welcome refuge from a harsh world. Some families are reluctant to come to the project initially as they do not want to be reminded of the bereavement, and are persuaded by the ease of access and flexibility we offer. Transport can be provided for families if needed, which is greatly appreciated. Travelling around South London with a young family is not easy, and families without a car find St Christopher's Hospice hard to access by public transport. The welcome starts with the greeting from the St Christopher's volunteer driver, and continues through reception and the overall impression of peaceful purposefulness in the hospice. Candle project staff need to engage with families immediately to ensure that they return for the next session. Both a warm welcome and a clear description of what Candle can offer are required to create the good working alliance necessary for any successful therapeutic intervention (Clarkson 1995). The working alliance, in our context, can be defined as the element of the counselling that persuades the family to keep attending for sessions even when sessions are experienced as painful or difficult. Critical to the creation of the alliance is the trustworthiness and ability of the counsellor, as perceived by the family. The reputation of the Hospice and the fact that it has been caring for bereaved families for over 35 years provides a good basis for trust even before families arrive and workers add their own individual professional style to that base. The same factors that facilitate the creation of a productive therapeutic relationship can also easily promote dependency in people who are vulnerable through bereavement, and we have learned that the ending of the working relationship has to be in mind from the first session and the worker has to mention this from the outset.

Families are told in the first session that the work is short term, up to six sessions, but that they can come back if additional bereavement related issues arise. At this point most families do not take in most of this, and we need to repeat it in succeeding sessions. Asking a child if they can tell you how many times they have come and reminding them how many more sessions they have is one way to help worker and client to focus. It often helps to plan a review with the child in the penultimate or final session. This is a way to affirm the child's learning and progress, and focuses attention on the end of the work. In the first year of the Candle project I was sometimes very anxious about ending after only six sessions with a child, only to have them tell me in the fifth meeting that they thought they had done it all really and were ready to move on. Six sessions, which may be spread over two or three months for various practical reasons, is a long time to a child. Sessions often follow the dates of school terms and come to a natural end with the end of term.

Team members often bring issues about the way that work is progressing to supervision and sometimes have to decide that some issues are not suitable for a short-term contract. One example was of a child who was in foster care and was told about a change of carer, which she then mentioned to the Candle worker. The child and the Social Services Department were keen that we took on the work of helping her through the change. Telling a child that you cannot work with her when she has shown her trust in you by opening the subject up is painful for any therapist and is a powerful argument for the importance of supervision as a space to look at the intense feelings that arise when working with children.

This example illustrates the importance of setting boundaries around the work of the project, and being clear about aims. The aim in this instance is 'to provide individual or group bereavement support to children young people and families in South East London bereaved by death' (Candle leaflet 1998). We do not offer support to families who are experiencing loss that is not through death as our area of expertise from our base in palliative care is bereavement by death. Attempting to be all things to all children merely dilutes the expertise that we do possess, and places unsustainable demands on our resources. In this situation we persuaded the Social Services Department to allocate a support worker to the child to help her with the change of carer.

Children need concrete reminders of a piece of short-term work to enable them to hold on to their memories of us as well as the reason they attended. All agencies develop their own techniques in this area. At the Candle project we take a Polaroid picture of the staff member together with the child, which they keep to remember our work together. We also give them a St Christopher's bear, one of the small mascots provided by the fund-raising department, and a badge. We might remind a young child that they can talk to Christopher bear when they need to, or at times when they would have talked to us. The ending is deliberately ritualized and sometimes tearful, but the message is always positive. We believe that the child can and will cope, and we give them many affirming messages both during the sessions and when we say goodbye.

How do we convey the invitation to return?

The family may be told several times about the possibility of coming back. The first may be over the phone if they ask for details and they will certainly be told on first assessment meeting. We have found that, as with most of the information we provide, this information needs to be repeated. Bereaved families have so much to think about and bereavement affects concentration. In the last session we address the issue of coming back directly, even if the topic has been discussed previously. The balance must be maintained between the offer of on-going support, made because we recognize that life continues to be hard for bereaved families, and the positive message of encouragement and belief in the family's ability to cope. Each of us will have our own form of words. I usually say something like, 'This is our last session, but I want you to know that if something comes up that reminds you about daddy's death and that he is not here for you, and you feel that you need to come and see me again then you must tell mummy and we will arrange it. I am going to tell mummy this too'. I then ask them if they can think of any examples of times they might need to see me again. Some children are very aware of these times and answer immediately, others may need some suggestions, but always as possibilities, to leave the choice of returning with the child. 'Maybe around your next birthday or when the anniversary of the death comes round. Some children find it hard at those times, not all need to come back but some do.' I then repeat this to the parent with the child there, so the invitation is for both of them. This contextualizes the message for parents and children, and parents sometimes make a note to make contact at those times to talk things through. The extended warranty can be accessed by families through telephone contact alone and we always encourage families to telephone us if they want to discuss issues, however trivial or unrelated they may feel these issues are.

What are the limitations to the warranty?

The obvious limitation is relevance. Families in need will approach the agencies that delivered help the last time and will make contact about issues that have little or no connection with the bereavement. Our approach is to talk through the issue initially over the telephone and then discuss in supervision if it seems to fall outside the parameters of the 'bereavement related issues' included in the warranty. Sometimes the phone call is sufficient, which highlights the importance of an accessible telephone service. This is described in more detail in Chapter 7. Many of the calls taken by Candle are from concerned parents or professionals who want to talk through their anxieties with someone they believe has greater expertise than they have. Parents who have a relationship with us will often call to seek reassurance or ideas about a situation that is worrying them and are then empowered to take action without the need for a meeting. Clear, sensible advice which can be accessed without the possibility of stigmatizing the child is of enormous value to many parents (Levy 2004).

A parent called the project because her teenage son was having difficulties at school. He had enjoyed his sessions two years previously at Candle and she wondered if he could be seen again as she thought that his difficulties might be linked to the death of his father several years ago. Looking at the notes, the worker at the time had commented that he enjoyed the sessions, especially playing games, but had not wanted to talk about his father with whom he had never had a close relationship as his parents had separated soon after his birth. Her feeling had been that the issue was his relationship with his mother who did not feel happy with his placement in a school for children with learning difficulties. At that time his mother agreed that she found it difficult to parent her son and was intending to seek counselling for herself. When she referred him again to the project, the original staff member had left and another worker agreed to see him for an assessment. She felt that the issue was still that of his relationship with his mother and that there was no sense of a bereavement reaction to his father's death.

This example highlights the importance of having a clear sense of purpose for the project and of providing opportunities for staff to reflect and discuss all the issues that arise when working in this emotionally intense area. Staff at Candle receive regular individual supervision from their manager and group supervision following every groupday.

The other limitation to the warranty is that of timing. Issues that arise years after the death are more likely to be unrelated, but families may need and appreciate the chance to discuss things over the phone or in person.

A parent with a long relationship with the project asked for her daughter, now aged 10, to be seen as her behaviour had changed recently and she had become very quiet and withdrawn. Her mother wondered if this could be due to a delayed grief reaction. Her father had died six years before, and the child had not been seen at the time as her mother did not feel she needed to, although her older brother, who was then 10, had been seen. The Candle worker met with the child as she would not talk to her mother at all. In the meeting, although she said very little, the issue was clearly not bereavement related, and the staff member felt that her preoccupation was probably due to her anticipation of the approaching move to secondary school. She fed this back to the parent, who talked to her daughter and confirmed that this was the case.

Does the warranty apply if the staff member has left?

This does happen, and several families every year reaccess the service and are seen by a worker who is new to them. We always make it clear that the warranty is an agreement between the family and the project, not the individual worker. A staff member might feel for any number of reasons that they were not able to work with a family again, or that they would benefit from a change, and the same could apply to a family. The services of the project are also structured in a way that dilutes the attachment to an individual worker. Families are invited to attend a groupday, and their worker may not be part of that day. If parents attend the bereavement or self-help groups they will meet staff and volunteers previously unknown to them. Although this arrangement grew out of practical necessity in a small team, it is appropriate for an agency that aims to encourage families to use all help available to them and to expand their relationships as their confidence grows. At the first assessment meeting, we explain that we keep records of our work, and that these records are confidential within the staff team and available to the parent if they wish to see them. As with much of the information that we give to bereaved families, it is doubtful how much they remember, so we now produce a written piece of information as well. Sometimes we need to seek families' agreement to share some of this information with other agencies for their benefit, as in the following example:

A young girl, Susan, was seen by the project following the death of her maternal grandmother, who was also her carer. Her mother had had no contact with her for several years, and after his wife's death, her step-grandfather, Nicholas took on the responsibility of caring for her. Susan was offered individual sessions and attended a groupday with her carer. Several months later, Nicholas approached the project again as Susan's mother was requesting contact. He was unhappy about this, as when her mother had made contact in the past she had ended the arrangement abruptly and Susan had been confused and distressed. He was also worried that Social Services would grant custody to Susan's mother, as he was not her blood relative. The staff member they had worked with previously had left and Nicholas agreed to another project worker speaking to the Social Services on his behalf. When contacted, the social worker was very appreciative of the opportunity to discuss the issue, as she was looking for support for her decision to restrict contact with Susan's mother. The staff member wrote a formal letter to Social Services with a copy to Nicholas supporting his care of Susan and describing his involvement with the Candle project. Nicholas was reassured by Social Services that there was no question of losing custody of Susan.

Sometimes families will not want to see another worker, but we have found that most are more concerned about the help they need than who they get it from. If the family feel that the project as a whole, which includes all the parts of the hospice they come into contact with, has been part of their support system, they will be less likely to refuse a 'new' worker. The attachment will be to the institution, which includes the support services, volunteers and the wider physical and social environment. One parent told me that one of the reasons she valued the sessions for her children so much was the chance it gave her to sit in the dining room with a coffee and read while looking out at the garden, secure in the knowledge that her child was meeting with me. Time out for bereaved parents, however short, is a valuable commodity.

Who can refer back?

As with initial referral, anyone can refer, but of course the family has to agree to the referral. If the contact comes from a school or other agency, we make an initial phone call to the family to assess the current situation. The parent carer self-help group also makes referrals back to the project at times.

After the sudden death from illness of their father Alan, all three children in the family were seen by two different staff members at Candle. All attended groupdays, and their mother attended the ongoing parent carers group, which she found very helpful. Two years later, she talked in that group of the problems she had been having with her eldest son, Sam, who was now 16 and had left home and was living in a hostel. Their relationship, which had not been happy since Alan's death (he had been much closer to his son), had broken down, and Marie was very distressed about it but unable to see a way through. The group facilitators encouraged her to make contact again with the staff of the project, and asked her if she would like them to contact us as well. Marie was glad of any help, but had felt that she should by now be managing independently. A meeting was arranged with her and her son, at which both aired their angry feelings. Although the meeting itself ended without resolution, they were able to talk afterwards and come to an understanding which allowed Sam to have more contact with his family.

Structuring the work

All re-referrals have to be considered and assessed and the system works because the numbers are not large. About 12–15% of families are referred back every year. The work is interesting for staff and is often a welcome change to meet again with a child or family further down the road. Families that come back are often very rewarding to work with as they have experienced the value of bereavement intervention. When families are seen again, only one or two sessions are offered. The main content of the work has been done and the issue prompting the recall can be dealt with in isolation. Children respond very well to this frame and often use the sessions to look at strategies for coping with difficult situations.

Jane's older brother, Martin, died in a road traffic collision in the autumn and she attended the project the following spring term. Two weeks before his birthday in the summer holidays, she asked her parents if she could come and see the staff member again as she had something important to talk about. She was worried about how the birthday was going to be managed and wanted to talk this through with the worker. Together they came up with some ideas and Jane made a card for her brother. She felt able to talk to her parents directly following the session.

This is an illustration of the rewards of offering the extended warranty. Children like Jane learn fast and use brief counselling appropriately to consider options. Therapeutically, the question arises of how much to focus on the 'here and now' issues and how much on the 'there and then' of the bereavement. This is best illustrated by a description of work done with a family who drew on the extended warranty many times in the four years of their contact with Candle. In this example, I have asked special permission from this family to tell their story in detail, and have only changed their names. In all other examples in the chapter I have used a number of methods to maintain anonymity.

Barry's father Dave died in a collision on his motor bike in July 1999. He was on holiday with a friend, and the collision happened when he came off his bike on a bend in the road and was thrown onto an oncoming car. His neck was broken and he died instantly. His wife Carrie stayed up all night after hearing the news from the police, waiting to tell Barry the news.

Barry was five and a half and his sister Mary was two and a half when I first met the family in November 1999. Barry was a very bright and articulate child with a reading ability well above the normal range, and he was very close to his father. Barry was finding it hard to talk about his father and was having difficulties with temper tantrums that he found hard to control, which made him an easy target for teasing at school. His mother was also seeing a bereavement counsellor, which made it easier for Barry to accept his need for counselling. He used the six sessions well to talk about the good memories he had of his father, and Carrie felt that he had been able to open up more.

In March the following year Barry attended a groupday for children which he enjoyed very much although he was the youngest child present. In July his mother referred him back to the project, as he had been very upset around the anniversary of the death. He had chosen to go to the school fete rather than attend a picnic with the other families from the Candle project and Carrie wondered if he had half expected to see his dad at the fete, as they had gone together the year before. Barry was very young when his father died, and it was quite possible that he did not fully understand the permanence of death. His immaturity was easy to miss, as he was so articulate and assured with adults. When we met he admitted that he had hoped to see his dad at the fete and we discussed the scientific reasons that people cannot come back from the dead, touched on the resurrection of Jesus, and asked one of the St Christopher's doctors how the paramedics would have checked to see that Dave was actually dead. Barry then told me that he knew anyway that people could not come back as he was very clever. (I have had some of the most difficult existential discussions of my professional career with bereaved children. They often demand to know my opinions and beliefs about issues I myself struggle with. I have always tried hard to be as honest as I can, although this has not always been the most comfortable answer for the child or for me.)

Barry also told me in this meeting that he wanted mum to find another dad, that he would be nice to him whoever he was, as long as he looked like Barry. We discussed the uniqueness of his relationship with his dad, and when I spoke to Carrie she told me that her husband's best friend Sam was now spending a lot of time with her and the children. Although she felt it was too early to think about a relationship, she could see that Barry was ahead of her.

The next contact came in November that year, when Barry asked to see me as he had become very upset as he realized that his father would not be there for Christmas. This had not really registered with him in the first year as things were still very recent, and the family were preoccupied with a planned trip to Australia which happened just after Christmas. This year Barry was very angry that his dad would not be there to do all the things with him that the other children's fathers were doing. He drew a picture of a Christmas tree with decorations for everyone in the family including his father, and we talked about feelings for people who had died being very powerful at Christmas.

Barry, as with several of the children we worked with, was upset about the events of September 11th 2001. Children who experienced the sudden death of a parent or close relative were reminded and distressed by the television footage of the sudden and traumatic deaths of so many other parents, and found themselves revisiting their own early reactions. Shortly after the attacks, his mother was due to attend a reception at the House of Commons with the Candle project parents' group, and Barry was very anxious about her attending. Carrie talked to him about the extra security there would be in that particular building and offered not to go if he was still worried. He thought it through and agreed to her attending.

In the spring of 2002 I saw Barry again as he wanted to talk about missing his dad, who was not there to tell him stories of what he had been was like when he was Barry's age. This is an example of the way in which a young child (he was still only 7) gradually realizes the many different aspects of bereavement. I could only agree with him that it was hard to have to accept this, and say that I was sorry that it hurt. We discussed how he could ask Sam about his father, as he had been friends with him since childhood. Barry said that it was very nice to have Sam around, but not as good as dad.

In 2003 Carrie told me that she and Sam and the children had decided to move to Australia. The children were excited, but did not fully understand that the distances would mean saying goodbye to their friends. She had been attending the parents group since it began, and was sad to be leaving them as well. We arranged a final session in July to say goodbye.

The whole family came for what was a very emotional session. Barry told me that he felt leaving his home, which was very linked for him with his father, would be hardest for him and for Sam. Sam was the one most like his father, and Sam had known him for so long. He told me again how he had been told the news of his father's death and cried, and how he had kept a bit of his motorbike and that when he grew older he would buy the same sort of bike. He said the person he would miss most was one friend at school who reminded him a lot of his father, and ended by telling me that his father had been the best father anyone could have had, and that 'the bond was going to be broken, but not too badly.' I was struck by his resourcefulness as he described ways he would hold on to memories, and his maturity as he talked about his link with his father.

Carrie had found the whole process leading up to the move very painful, as she was facing so many reminders. When her husband died she had not bothered to change the name on the television licence, and when she called to cancel it was told that she would have to send in a copy of his death certificate. This year, for the first time, Barry had forgotten to make a card for Fathers' Day, and Mary had made one for Sam and asked him to be her father. Carrie found this very difficult, as she herself was struggling with wanting to make a new life and move on but fearing that they would forget all that the old life had meant.

The family have now been in Australia for six months, and Carrie has emailed me regularly to update me on their progress. It has not been easy, but they are all still very positive and the children are thriving.

The contact I had with this family over a number of years demonstrates the importance of a service that is speedily accessible when needed. Children need space to consider strategies to cope with the changing demands of their lives as they grow and develop. The adults around them need opportunities to contact a service that has been helpful in the past if issues arise that they need help with. The service is rarely used inappropriately and if it is the costs on staff time are small. Many families require only a telephone call. The knowledge that someone is available if necessary is in itself sufficient for some families, and allows them to make the decision about contact when they feel they really need it. Families appreciate the autonomy this gives them. The service Candle delivers is designed to promote the natural resilience in the families we see by emphasizing their strengths and their capacity to overcome adversity. Over the time of a family's contact with us that service will change in nature to respond to their changing circumstances. Given the appropriate support and a good helping of luck, a family will come through a bereavement strengthened by the experience and better able to cope with any other adversities that may arise.

References

Black D (2002). Bereavement. In: M Rutter, E Taylor (ed.) *Child psychiatry: modern approaches* 4th edn, pp. 299–308. Oxford: Blackwells.

Christ GH (2000). *Healing children's grief.* Oxford: Oxford University Press.

Clarkson P (1995). *The therapeutic relationship.* London: Whurr.

Levy J (2004). Unseen support for bereaved children. *Bereavement Care* **23**(2), 25–7.

St Christopher's Candle Project (1998). *Information Leaflet.* London: St Christopher's Hospice.

Stokes J, Wyer S, Crossley D (1997). The challenge of evaluating a child bereavement programme. *Palliative Medicine* **11**:179–90.

Worden JW (1996). *Children and grief: when a parent dies.* New York: The Guilford Press.

Chapter 9

Swampy ground: brief interventions with families before bereavement

Gillian Chowns

In a book about children's bereavement this chapter is the odd one out, because its focus is on working with children *before* a death. Nevertheless the principles underpinning the work will no doubt be familiar to many readers, and these will be illustrated through a variety of case examples.

The context

Pre-bereavement work has to contend with one major and unique issue—uncertainty. However tragic the experience of a bereaved child, she knows where she is, she knows she is bereaved, and that someone important has died. This also applies to the worker. But supporting children in a family where a parent or grandparent is seriously ill, is like wading through a swamp that has been sown with land mines. There is precious little solid ground. What there is, may be likely to blow up in our face. We cannot always be certain of the outcome—is this father going to respond to treatment; is it realistic to think in terms of 'cure'? And if not, we still do not know how long he will survive, and therefore how long we may have to work with the child. So judging how we should pace our work is difficult. We may have just a few days, or perhaps several months; we do not know whether our first visit will also be the last or whether we will see child or parent or both maybe half a dozen times. Nevertheless, as the following case studies demonstrate, effective intervention does not necessarily require long-term therapeutic work. While our work usually reflects the experience of the sick person—that there is never enough time—it also reflects another truth of palliative care: that it is perfectly possible to make a difference even when time is limited, and often precisely *because* time is limited. The Broad family typified this.

Mum was already seriously ill, and deteriorating almost daily, when I first met her and her husband. It seemed likely that there might be a month or so to work with their two daughters, aged eight and ten, and I planned the first session accordingly, aiming to establish some rapport and trust, to explain who I was and how I might help, and to offer them some choice about whether and how we might work together. I also hoped to clarify both what they *knew* and *felt* about their mother's illness. The visit went well and I felt I had achieved or was working towards most of the objectives. I was then able to formulate a clear plan for the next visit. But it was postponed because Mum was admitted to the local hospice that day. She died a week later and my plan was obsolete. (That is not to say that plans aren't useful, just that we must always be willing to amend or abandon them in the light of the situation that presents itself rather than the one that we have anticipated.) Nevertheless, the foundation stones of the work were in place, even though the focus had shifted from supporting the children through their mother's illness to offering bereavement support. The girls—and their Dad—knew that help was available, that they could choose when and how to access it, and that the meaning that their loss had for them would be recognized and respected. Thus, although the referral had left us very little time to work together, it had still been possible to establish the core conditions of trust, respect, and choice for an effective intervention.

- ◆ Establish trust
- ◆ Check understanding as well as knowledge
- ◆ Offer options and agree a possible way forward

Pace, level, and age

In contrast, Alison Sellars confounded everyone by outliving her prognosis by many months. There were both positive and negative outcomes from this.

When I met her children, they were each struggling with the roller-coaster that was their mother's illness. Stuart, who had behavioural difficulties and was a weekly boarder at a Special School, was 14 and his sister Emma, bright and articulate, was 11. So the nature of my work with her was different from that with Stuart. She needed information about the disease, its consequences, and outcomes, but she also needed the opportunity to debate its implications for her—coming up to puberty, self-conscious about her developing breasts, and only too well aware of her mother's mastectomy. A number of our conversations were essentially debates about body image, although we did not use that language. Work with Stuart was much more task-oriented, concrete, and present rather than future-focused. Nevertheless, Stuart was a shrewd observer of his family and had a more realistic understanding of the situation than either parent realized. Shortly after I had begun work with the children, there was an explosive family row, when Dad lost control and shouted, 'Don't you know she's going to die? Stuart was able to give a good account of what that meant. 'I know she's ill and she won't get better and she'll go on getting iller, but it isn't like she's going to die tomorrow or next week, it could be a month or more'. His basic understanding was good, his emotions and behaviour much less mature. On the four or five occasions

I met with him, either at home or at his boarding school, I consciously tried to pitch my approach largely—though not exclusively—at his emotional age. Often angry at life, he frequently complained that 'it's not fair', and I was able to use this as a *motif* for our work. Although the concept of fairness was an abstract, we could work together on what was fair to expect from each member of the family. Used to a system of rewards and punishments, Stuart was comfortable with the idea of negotiating a 'fair' contract with his family about how much he helped around the house, how much special time he got with his mother and how frequently he could ring to check on things at home during his weekly absence. A week was a long time in his life and I needed to adjust my approach accordingly. With Emma, I could work more swiftly and reflectively, recognizing that she was much older than eleven most of the time, but that occasionally she needed and wanted to be more like a seven year old! Thus the pace of the work tried to take into account the children's (multiple) ages. But it also needed to take into account the likely dying trajectory (Pattison 1997) of their mother. Other concepts such as levels of awareness (Glaser and Strauss 1965) and anticipatory grief (Lindemann 1944) are also familiar and, usually, meaningful for professionals in planning and reviewing their work with a family. They may enable us to face the uncertainty that both the family and we experience. But the reality for Stuart and Emma was that they went to school each day not knowing whether their mother would still be at home in the afternoon, or whether she would have had another fall and another hospital admission. They knew their mother would die soon, but after every crisis she was still there. It became hard for them to live in this limbo. For them, those last few months were an eternity. They didn't know what 'anticipatory grief' meant, but they knew that both they and their Dad were finding it harder to be close to Alison. For that chronologically brief but emotionally extended period, it was important that the worker did not model that detachment and distance but demonstrated a willingness to stay with them in their pain, listen to their anger and acknowledge their weariness and fear. When uncertainty and exhaustion combine, the reliable presence of someone genuine, warm, and empathic (Egan 1990) can be a useful, short-term, counterbalance.

- ◆ Emotional maturity may be more important than chronological age.
- ◆ Identify and work with the child's concerns, at the child's intellectual level.
- ◆ Being (there) may be as important as doing.

Ethical issues

Short-term interventions are liable to criticism from two quarters. Some would argue that effective intervention requires sustained, long-term, intensive work. From others there have been criticisms in recent years of the grief and counselling 'industries', with Walter (1994) characterizing its proponents as 'grief police', peddling a one-size-fits-all approach, inappropriate for a post-modern society, and others suggesting that interventions may do more harm than good. Yet there is increasing evidence that skilled short-term work before a death can be beneficial for both child and family. Writers such as Jewett (1994) and Christ (2000) offer a sound theoretical base for practice. And the user-empowerment movement, with its drive for 'meaningful participation and consultation' (Monroe and Oliviere 2003: vi) is beginning to enable children (a largely marginalized group to date) to be heard. Although, in comparison with bereavement, there are still relatively few services for the about-to-be bereaved, and even less research on the topic, the situation has changed significantly in recent years.

Children's rights

It is a curious fact that, in Western society at least, there is a deep ambivalence about children. We have extended the period of childhood, in terms of education and economic dependence, into the late teens; yet we have also shortened it drastically, as we turn childhood into a consumer experience and target children as mini-adults, selling them life-style and success through the latest 'must-have' trainers, clothes, or computer games. We are both pro- and anti-children in almost equal measure. On the one hand, we see them as innocent, vulnerable, and in need of protection, and on the other hand, we see them as dangerous—hanging round on street corners, out of control, and in need of discipline and containment (Beresford 2002).

Alongside this ambivalence, however, can be discerned a clear trend to recognize children as individuals and, indeed, citizens in their own right, and as a consequence, *with* their own rights. The Children Act 1989 emphasized the 'best interests' of the child as 'paramount', and enshrined a child's right to refuse consent to medical examinations and assessments. More significant in theory, but perhaps less so in practice, was another 1989 piece of legislation, the UN Declaration of the Rights of the Child. Articles 12 and 13 clearly set out the right of a child to be informed, consulted, and involved in any 'matters which affect their well-being'. For the first time, and applicable to all cultures, there was a public, global acknowledgement that children should not only be seen but also be heard—that they are capable of forming their own views and that those views must be considered carefully. Within the UK context, this issue had been hotly contested through the courts in the Gillick case. Fundamentally concerned with consent and competence in relation to contraception services, the case attracted much media attention. The House of Lords judgement strengthened children's rights and weakened parents', in that it ruled that a young person under 16 was capable of deciding for herself about contraception, and that a professional, in this case the GP, did not have to obtain parental consent to provide a service. While later case law has muddied the waters somewhat (BMA 2002), this was undoubtedly a landmark ruling, confirming that a minor's views about her own needs were privileged over a parent's wish to control or protect.

By the beginning of the new millennium, the principle that children were capable of forming their own views, potentially competent to decide what was right for them, and entitled to have those views heard and respected, was well established. This provides a fairly sound ethical basis for working with children who are facing the possible death of a parent. However, as in other social work settings, parental wishes and rights may conflict with those of the children. In the palliative care context the highly prized notion of patient autonomy is often a case in point.

Conflicting rights–parents who block

Mrs L was terminally ill with pancreatic cancer, but resisted all attempts by professionals to persuade her to tell her three children of eight, five, and three that she was not going to get better. The rights of the children to appropriate support, information, and involvement were all negated by her right to be 'in denial' (a much misused term, but almost certainly applicable in this instance), and her legal position as parent. In this situation, it was important to identify not what *should* be done, but what *could*, realistically be done, and to focus on that. So the aim of the work was necessarily more modest, but still valuable–to identify support networks for the children and father in the event of her death, and to liaise with these agencies, such as schools and health visitors, who were already, and would continue to be, involved with the children. Mrs L could accept the need for teachers and the Health Visitor to be involved 'while I'm ill' and was keen to have help with transport to school, and extra time at a nursery for Jodie, the three year old. Although it proved impossible to engage her in future plans for the family, we nevertheless had established a network of other professionals to support the family for reasons that she regarded as legitimate (education and health) rather than, in her view, the unacceptable one of terminal illness. Those networks would be just as relevant after her death, and would be able to sustain the family over a substantial period of time, if appropriate. Thus, two difficult but carefully negotiated sessions resulted in some positive outcomes for the children and their father, even though the mother appeared to be largely avoiding her children's needs.

- Identify support networks and mobilize 'acceptable' resources
- Focus on what could be done rather than on what should be done—aim to find some common ground.

Of course, it may also work the other way. Many parents will assure a worker that their child is keen to be seen, but it quickly emerges on a first visit that he has little understanding of who that worker is or what they do, and has been given no choice in the matter of meeting them. The parent's *need* to help their child, however well-intentioned, has overridden the child's *right* not only to consent but to give an *informed* consent to the meeting. In these situations, a pragmatic approach seems sensible.

Negotiating access

Mrs Mitchell, a divorced mother with breast cancer was asking for help with her teenage children. However, she admitted that her 14-year-old daughter was resistant to the idea of outside help.

All I had learnt strongly suggested that Leone was distressed and isolated—which distressed her mother—but how ethical was it to persist, in the light of her alleged reluctance?

Clearly, the mother was keen to have support. And as yet, the daughter had not personally refused help. On a follow-up visit, Leone was present, albeit reluctantly, I negotiated with her to have five minutes of her time, on the understanding that she did not have to do anything more than listen. I used the time to do three things—to explain my role, to emphasize that I would always respect confidentiality, and to make clear that the choice was entirely hers (not mine or her mother's) as to whether, when or how she used the help on offer. Faced with a teenager who exuded anger, fear, and confusion, it was tempting to try and do more, but it was important to demonstrate that I could be trusted to keep my word. Leone now knew that some help was available if she wanted it, that there was an adult who would respect her wishes and feelings, and that if she did not want to take up the offer now, she could always do so later. Respect, choice, and control were on offer in a way that was probably unfamiliar in this household that had apparently been a battleground between her two needy parents for so many years.

Establishing which other professionals were, or could appropriately be, involved and liaising with them was also crucial. Direct work with a child may not always be possible but if we have enabled family members and other professionals to agree access and involvement, then we may have done as much as we ethically should or could.

- Be clear about your role
- Respect a young person's right to reject help—but make clear that they can change their mind later
- Only make promises that you are able and prepared to keep

Firm foundations

Both social work and health care ethics require us to consider not only how we approach the work but to be clear about the theories which may or may not underpin what we do in the messy world of real practice.

The literature on childhood bereavement, while substantially less than the volume produced on adult bereavement, is nevertheless growing exponentially (Furman 1974; Dyregrov 1991; Worden 1991; Klass *et al.* 1996; Barnard *et al.* 1999). But pre-bereavement, to use my shorthand, is self-evidently not the same, for all of the reasons highlighted above. For many years there was very little writing and research on this, and the tendency was to fall back on the bereavement literature for guidance. By definition, this is retrospective—even when the interviews focus on life before the parent died, the young person is recalling it as a past event with the benefit of hindsight, in full awareness that death was the outcome. Nevertheless, there is now a developing body of literature that focuses on living with (anticipated) loss (Black and Wood 1989; Jewett 1994; Sheldon 1997; Christ 2000; Kissane and Bloch 2000). Some studies have focused more particularly on communication issues (Barnes *et al.* 2000; Landry-Datteé and Delaigue-Cosset 2001), but there are relatively few large scale studies of children facing the possible death of a parent. However, Christ's work, which researched families both pre- and post-death, offers a comprehensive, thoughtful, and structured approach to working with anticipated death, which identifies the psychological, developmental stages as key to understanding the child's needs, responses, and coping strategies.

The growth of this area of research is good news, for it has been tempting to think that the previous dearth of research mirrored the practice situation—that professionals found this area 'scary'. There may be three reasons for this. First, its very uncertainty— its 'swampy' nature—makes *us* uncertain of our abilities and skills. Secondly, the combination of children and death is both powerful and disabling. We instinctively reject it as not natural; it challenges our notions of fair play, and the innocence of childhood. Our instinct, like that of so many parents, is to protect the children—and possibly ourselves. We fear making things worse. Just as many parents from the best of motives avoid talking to their children about such painful issues, so many researchers may have avoided this area for the same reasons. Ethical concerns about intruding on grief, raising levels of anxiety, and making children fear the worst may be understandable or even legitimate, but the consequence is that they have been marginalized and disempowered; their voice is not heard. Thirdly, the area may just be too close to home. Staying alongside the distress of children is difficult; it confronts us with both our own remembered childhood and also with our own mortality—another uncomfortable combination.

For these, and maybe other reasons, pre-bereavement groups such as my own team's 'Video Project', a closed group of nine youngsters who met weekly to make a video of their own experiences, are much rarer than bereavement groups such as the well-established Winston's Wish, Daisy's Dream, or Stepping Stones, with their residential weekends, reunions, or regular sessions. The welcome increase in pre-bereavement research may encourage practitioners to redress the balance somewhat.

What else may we draw upon? Two other resources suggest themselves. The social work and sociological literature on families can be helpful (Walsh and McGoldrick 1991; Walsh 1993) as an earlier chapter has already demonstrated. Any social work student worth his salt knows that change and loss are enduring themes in the work, whether it is with elderly clients facing physical deterioration and possible institutional care, the mentally ill facing loss of freedom and identity, the adoptive couple facing the loss of reproductive identity even as they gain a baby, or children in the care system losing family, home, and school all at once (Jewett 1994). Palliative care, a particularly specialized area of change and loss, can usefully draw upon and contribute to the social work literature available. Within this, the literature on counselling children (Geldard and Geldard 1997; Barwick 2000) is relevant. Much that Geldard and Geldard have to say, particularly about the goals of counselling and active listening, is transferable, even though their context is specifically psychotherapeutic. More broadly, while the finality of death is qualitatively different from all the other crises with which they, other psychotherapists, school counsellors, and youth workers deal, the issues of identity, uncertainty, choice, and control remain central.

Counselling in general, and bereavement support in particular have been strongly criticized in more recent years and palliative care itself is vulnerable to the charge that there is no evidence base for its effectiveness. Part of the problem, of course, is agreeing what constitutes an evidence-base. Whether it is either feasible or desirable to apply positivistic notions of measurement to the individual kaleidoscope of experiences, meanings, and values that make up a child's journey through life is debatable. But the work highlighted above offer some useful models and theories that provide a solid foundation for our work; they can, as Christ (2000) suggests, guide, though not prescribe, our interventions. As we also continue to reflect both on, and in, action (Schon 1987) we too can build on those foundations.

However, a *caveat* is called for. Just as history is partial because it is written by the (generally male) winners, so is the research basis for intervention with children partial. We still await the definitive version, written by those who have lived it–the children. It may be that, as Alderson (1995) and Barnard *et al.* (1999) have suggested, children are not simply passive recipients of skilled adult professional intervention, but that they are active participants in their own lives, marshalling their own peer-based support networks, seeking out and processing information, selecting strategies and, essentially exercising control. So, while we should be encouraged by the development of a more solid, research-based foundation to justify our work, we need to hold on to a certain humility. We are not the all-powerful *deus ex machina* working on the blank canvas of another human being, but are subject to social, political, and cultural contexts and ultimately to the main actor, the child, who will herself judge whether she needs or wants to work with us. Sensitive, qualitative research has begun to articulate something of the child's voice, but there is room for more collaborative, user-involved research to enable the child's voice to take centre-stage.

Brief interventions in the family home

The following stories typify some of the challenges and opportunities faced by practitioners working in the community setting—which usually means in the family's home. They demonstrate a range of interventions over a relatively brief period of time— sometimes days, sometimes a few months–that were underpinned by the principles of honesty, respect, choice, and control.

Helping parents to help their children

The Andrews family had been impressive in their willingness to face the likely loss of Martin, Dad to Jenny and Todd and husband to Elaine. Now that Martin was deteriorating noticeably, Elaine was, typically, anxious to think ahead to what would happen when he died. She wondered if she should send the children away to her Mum 'when it gets really close'.

She thought it might be sensible to get the children back into school as soon as possible after the death, as 'it would be better than hanging round the house'. She supposed that Jenny, aged seven, was too young to go to the funeral, but that Todd, at nine, was probably old enough. She was a little surprised by the question 'What do Jenny and Todd think?' but it provoked a fruitful discussion, in which I highlighted the very sensitive way she had responded to their different needs and understandings so far, and how consistent she had been in checking out at each stage how much they understood, how much they wanted to know, and how involved they wanted to be in Martin's care. Her child-centred approach had worked well to date, so maybe there was no need to change it now. Elaine was able to admit, somewhat ruefully, that she had uncharacteristically not considered the children's wishes. Our discussion then moved on to ways of raising these issues with the children, but was interrupted by the arrival of Todd in the sitting room. In a three-way conversation between us, Todd revealed how he was worried about being teased at school because 'When Dad dies, they will call me a bastard, 'cos I won't have a Dad any more'. Between us, Elaine and I were able to help Todd work out a plan. Todd thought he himself would want to tell his best friend when his Dad died, but that he would like his class teacher to tell the class—'but when I'm not there'. A question about who he might want to talk to, if he got very upset, elicited the answer, 'Mrs Taylor', the class helper. Later, after I'd left, Elaine was able to have a similar conversation with Jenny, who was much less certain about what she wanted. The discussion with Todd, however, had enabled Elaine to suggest some options to Jenny, so that together they agreed an acceptable plan. On my next visit, Elaine was keen to tell me how supportive the school had been when she had contacted them. She was pleased and relieved to have a plan in place—but quickly acknowledged that the children might easily change their minds when it came to the actual event. She could apply the same *caveat* to the discussion she was planning to have with them about attending the funeral. She was no longer so focused on protecting them from what she had thought would be an unsuitable and distressing experience. She now wanted to support them, and was able to recognize their right to be involved, if that was their choice. Involvement, to her, had meant simply attending, but as she talked about what Martin wanted (cremation) and the hymns he had chosen in advance, I was able to ask the same basic question again, 'What will Todd and Elaine want (to contribute)?' Although Elaine did not feel strong enough to talk in detail about the funeral with the children at this stage, the fact that we had been able to think through the issues meant that when Martin eventually died the children were involved and included as much as they wanted to be. Both of them chose to put a favourite item in the coffin; each had a suggestion for some music to be played during the ceremony, and a memory about their Dad that the minister could share with the congregation. Todd was clear that he not only wanted to go to the funeral but that he wanted to see his father's body at the undertaker's. Jenny was less sure; she said she would go with the others, but she wouldn't go in and see the body. Elaine said that was fine, and that Grandma would wait with her outside the room. In the event, Jenny surprised them by electing to go in just as they were ready to leave. Elaine followed the same principle with the funeral; taking account of the children's wishes, but offering the option for them to change their minds right up until the service itself. This time, she had prepared a cousin of hers, well-known to the children, to go with them if either became so distressed that they didn't want to stay. The fact that (at some emotional cost to herself) she had taken them both to the crematorium a few days before the funeral and had painstakingly explained what happened in the service, including when the coffin would disappear behind the curtains, meant that both Todd and Jenny were better able to cope; they both stayed throughout the service. Elaine faced some criticism from some of her relatives but was sustained by Todd's comment, 'All those other people were there, but they weren't family like we are, I needed to be there for Dad'.

The importance of memories

In the weeks before Martin's death, the children and I had talked about some of the special memories they had of their Dad. Sometimes it was a family outing that they recalled, sometimes it was a mannerism of his, or a saying he was fond of. Some of these 'favourite things' were captured in the workbook that Jenny and I used, but Todd had not wanted to do one. Using his computer for the same end, however, worked very well. Todd liked lists, and was happy to compile a long list of all his Dad's favourite things–food, colours, TV programmes, etc. After Martin died, the workbook and the computer file served as prompts for Todd and Jenny, enabling them to hold on to precious memories. While some of the adults around them avoided Martin's name, as if he had never existed, the children had their own treasure store which they could 'activate' as and when they needed.

It is not only memories that need preserving; for children, as for adults, possessions may carry a significance way beyond their material value. Children may be hesitant about asking for something belonging to the dying parent, so it may be helpful for the worker to raise the issue. For some families, a memory box in which significant items are kept has pride of place; for Todd, wearing his father's watch was all that mattered. As he confided in me, 'It smells of him, and that makes me sad, and happy'.

◆ Facilitate parent—child communication

◆ Challenge untested assumptions—gently!

◆ Encourage families to involve children in funeral plans—and respect their choices

◆ Make it clear that it is OK to change your mind at any time

◆ Find ways of preserving memories of the dead parent

Listening

Roy and David were teenage brothers whose mother was terminally ill. Their father contacted our team for support for them. Teenagers are generally recognized to be hard to engage, and boys more difficult than girls. So the combination of gender and age was not encouraging. In addition the first meeting in the family kitchen brought to the fore the issues of consent and ethics referred to earlier in the chapter. Neither of the boys had themselves requested to see me; it was their father who was instigating the referral. Clearly unable to resist his urgings, the boys agreed to a second visit. Offered the choice of being seen individually (my own private preference) or together, they chose the latter. In the end, I had two sessions with them before their mother died. I began by suggesting that, although I knew the main facts from their father, they might like to tell me the story in their own words. And that's what they did. What *I* did, almost exclusively, was to listen. The value of this simple 'narrative' approach was threefold. First, it enabled them, perhaps as never before, to put the pieces together, to establish a chronology and to make some limited sense of events. Second, it enabled them to articulate some of their beliefs and meanings about the experience. Thirdly, they were able to explore, challenge, and build on each other's differing memories, perceptions, and concerns. Contrary to all the family's expectations, 14 year old David was almost as vocal as his more confident brother of 16. Both he and Roy admitted to being surprised about this, while I wondered to myself whether David would have said anything at all if I had followed my own instincts and seen him separately!

In this situation the ability to listen, to offer some prompts (sparingly), to take the boys seriously, and to acknowledge in the beginning that they had some choices about how they used the help that they had not asked for, was sufficient. More than a year later, in response to a researcher's interview, they said, 'It was good doing it before [Mum died] rather than after ... it was in a big part of our brain, it was on our minds all the time. ... I wasn't as upset when she actually died as I thought I would be because I had come to terms with it then, and if I had the counselling after ... I might have been more upset'. So gender and age are important—but not insuperable!

- ◆ Listening to the story is often the most important thing we do
- ◆ Acknowledge that everyone will experience the story differently—there is no one truth

Rehearsing, informing, and ignoring

Differentiation is an important precept in educational circles, equally applicable in working in palliative care, as Christ (2000) makes abundantly clear, and never more so than when working with siblings.

Michael, Rosie, and Lesley were eleven, nine, and seven when I first met them, at the request of their Mum whose cancer had begun to spread.

Michael was a sensible, mature child with some understanding of what was happening and some questions for which he needed honest answers. After two sessions he decided he didn't need any more help but thought that his sisters still did. He had sufficient information for his current needs and did not want anything more, at that stage. I discovered that he related well to his Year Head and his Head Teacher, trusted them both and felt able to talk to them easily. He did not need another adult support; he had already identified some adults who would be available for him. His behaviour supports Christ's observations of the developmental needs of this age group—a preference for factual information and a reluctance to engage in emotional exploration.

Rosie (9) was thirsty for attention, always had lots to tell and lots to ask, and was able to be quite open about her worries. One particular session stands out. I knew her Mum was worried about Rosie; that she was finding school difficult, and equally that the school were concerned. Almost certainly Rosie was frightened about the future. I arranged to pick her up from school and take her out to tea. As we munched away at our mega-burgers, Rosie relaxed, and after a hesitant start, poured out her worries. She was concerned that her Mum tried to do too much: 'she goes out Monday and does shopping and loads of stuff and she wants to get things done and not stop, and then on Tuesday she can't do nothing, she's so tired and I think, then if she goes on like that the cancer will come back'. She was worried, too, about her Dad's smoking; 'I know it causes cancer, I wish he would stop but he doesn't listen, I'm afraid he might get cancer and die'. She was finding it hard to cope with home and school and felt overwhelmed by everything: 'I know they have got a lot on their plate, but *my* plate's full, it's overflowing'. We had a long talk about these worries and how she could share them with her parents, but Rosie was convinced it would be too difficult – 'Could you do it, please?' Though my aim had been to empower her to do it, I finally agreed. I dropped her back home, promising to phone to make an appointment to see her Mum. When I rang the next day, Mum told me how distressed Rosie had been on her return from tea with me. Then she explained how Rosie had poured out all her worries, including her fear that Mum—and Dad if he continued smoking—would die. Mum had sat Rosie on her lap and they had cried together. 'It feels so much better' said Mum. 'We had a really good talk and I've been as honest as I can with her.'

So I never needed to make that particular appointment. Rehearsing her fears, and rehearsing what she wanted to be said (by me on her behalf) enabled Rosie to go and do it herself.

Lesley was a real contrast to Rosie. Apparently placid and 'no trouble', she did not cause her parents any particular worries. But they wanted to be fair to all their children and to do the best for them—so they were keen that Lesley should not be left out. Mum and Dad believed that it was good to talk, so they were insistent that all three siblings should not only see me but talk to me. As often happens, parental needs were in conflict with children's wishes. Lesley and I resolved this by meeting together with her brother and sister for a fun session of painting and drawing that was messy, relaxed, and yet productive on two levels. For Lesley it provided a safe space, away from the tensions of home, where she could genuinely relax, without the need to contribute to discussions or openly acknowledge her feelings. However, the card she chose to make for her mother was a very concrete statement of her feelings. It was something visible, and personal, a gift that she could give, but that had not required painful verbal communication. She had been in control of the activity and in the process of spreading glue, glitter and gum all over the room, she had occasionally offered apparently casual or unrelated asides that clearly indicated her underlying thoughts. I chose to acknowledge each of these but not to pursue them if Lesley did not respond. Although the literature is right to emphasize the benefits of open discussion, it is not what every child always wants. Lesley was well aware that her mother was going to die, but it was her choice to ignore it most of the time. It would be easy but wrong to label this as denial. All of us are well able to hold two inconsistent positions at once. For example, we know the exam is approaching, but we don't get down to revision; we need to lose weight, but we have just one last cake – again! Lesley's coping strategy was to be determinedly cheerful and to avoid talking about the inevitable. In this, also, she was her father's child. She had always been less ready to talk, so why should cancer in the family make her more ready? Ignoring the problem (most of the time) worked for Lesley (most of the time), and I needed to respect that. And having fun for fun's sake, was important for all these siblings. A common thread in all the literature is the nature of children's grief – powerful but intermittent – and the need for normality. On both counts, the opportunity to be a child and to do normal, child-like things, was valuable/therapeutic.

- Clear information is important
- A safe space to practise what to say can encourage children to communicate directly with parents
- Not everyone needs to talk. But all children need to still be able to have fun

Expert knowledge

Specialized knowledge in terms of either the illness or normal childhood development and behaviour is almost a 'given' in our work. However, other areas of expertise may be helpful in their own right—and serve as an entry point for more intense, emotionally oriented work.

> The Chana family wanted expert, practical advice about securing the children's future after Mum's death. She was divorced from her husband and the children, aged 18 and 14 lived, very happily it seemed, with her. The son saw his father occasionally; the daughter never. Mother and daughter were adamant that they did not want the father to have any role in the children's future, let alone any parental power or responsibility. That, however, was just what he would have on her death, as the sole person *in loco parentis*. This family had not asked for counselling or emotional support, but for help with what they defined as their most urgent task. The intervention was brief—to ascertain the legal situation, give information about guardianship and other options, highlight some of the issues to be considered, and then leave the family to make up their own minds. The facts that I had given them enabled them to plan for the future, make their own choices and gain some peace of mind. What was helpful to them was to have some sound advice about guardianship and the rights of parents and children, rather than an exploration of their inner feelings. However, once the practical problem was resolved, mother and daughter could acknowledge some of their emotions. In this case, supporting the family to deal with the practicalities enabled them to test out their worker. Reassured that I could be trusted over practical advice, and that they could choose their own pace, they were then able to risk sharing some of their emotional problems. A tentative reflection, 'You've been very clear about the practical issues but I'm just wondering whether all the feelings about what's happening are as easy to deal with?' led each of them to admit how worried they were about the other family members. When Amrit said she thought her brother was very scared even though he did not say so, I asked her what assumptions her brother might be making about her, and this moved the conversation on to a much more open discussion about her own emotions. It was important to work with their priorities, at their pace, but to be alert to the opportunity, when it was offered, to confront their own individual emotions.

- Prioritize—practical issues may be more pressing than emotional ones
- Only when a family feels secure about their future may they be able to explore their emotional insecurity.

Practising what we preach

Working with death and dying is demanding; so is working with children. Doing both at once is always going to be stressful. We do not help anyone if we assume a god-like immunity to stress.

Developing a sense of humour has been a traditional coping strategy, and has its uses; but if it becomes cynical, it may be time to take stock. We preach the need for quality of life to our clients, adult or child, patient or carer, but may be poor at applying it to ourselves. The importance of a life outside work hardly needs stating. Skilled supervision, something that social work has always recognized but that the NHS has been slower to embrace, is a *sine qua non*. We need, and our clients are entitled to expect us to have, an outside perspective on our work—someone who can both support and challenge us, who can identify the recurring themes in our work and who can give us what we try to give our clients–time, space, and value.

Supervision should also help us to accept our own limitations. Why should we expect to be equally skilled at working with teenagers as with two year olds? Why, if we are parents of a rebellious boy, should we be surprised to find ourselves sympathetic to the sick parent whose son seems intent on adding to his distress? There are times when it is sensible, safe, and professional to say: 'No - no, it's not wise for me to do this piece of work.'

Finally, we should remember that while detachment and objectivity are important, it is no sin to feel distress. A permanently prostrate professional is no earthly good to anyone, but if we cannot keep in touch with our own humanity, there is no hope for us or those we try to help.

Last words

Children whose parents are seriously ill present particular challenges. Their status in society is disputed; their competence and understanding undervalued. Their rights and needs are often in conflict with those of their parents. Their future is uncertain, for they do not know when they will join the ranks of the bereaved. Yet, effective work with these children rests on a few, well-known, simple precepts. Our role is not to become part of the problem by increasing their dependence on us, but rather genuinely to empower them to find their own way. In the video made by our own young people's group (Chowns *et al.* 2003), there is one clear message from all the children: 'Tell us the truth'. But there is another equally important message: 'Don't tell us that you know how we feel—you don't. We're all different'. We need to respect those differences. If we are able to hold on to those guiding principles of honesty and respect, choice and control, while honouring difference we shall stand a good chance of negotiating both the minefields and the swamp.

References

Alderson P (1995). *Listening to children.* Barkingside: Barnados.

Barnard P, Morland I, Nagy J (1999).*Children, bereavement and trauma.* London: Jessica Kingsley.

Barnes J, Kroll L, Burke O *et al.* (2000). Qualitative interview study of communication between parents and children about maternal breast cancer. *British Medical Journal* **321**:479–82.

Barwick N (2000). *Clinical counselling in schools.* London: Routledge.

Beresford P (2002). Maturity needed. *Community care* **July 11**, 20.

Black D, Wood D (1989). Family therapy and life-threatening illness in children or parents. *Palliative Medicine* **3**(2), 113–18.

British Medical Association (2001). *Consent, rights and choices in health care.* London: BMJ Books.

Chowns G *et al.* (2003). *No - you don't know how we feel* (Video). Windsor: East Berks Palliative Care Team.

Christ G (2000). *Healing children's grief.* New York: Oxford University Press.

Dyregrov A (1991). *Grief in children.* London: Jessica Kingsley.

Egan G (1990). *The skilled helper.* California: Brooks Cole Publishing.

Furman E (1974). *A child's parent dies.* New Haven, CT: Yale University Press.

Geldard K, Geldard D (1997). *Counselling children.* London: Sage.

Glaser B, Strauss A (1965). *Awareness of dying.* Chicago, IL: Aldine.

Jewett C (1994). *Helping children cope with separation and loss.* Boston: B.T. Battsford.

Kissane DW, Bloch S (2002). *Family focused grief therapy.* Buckingham: Open University Press.

Klass D, Silverman P, Nickman S (1996). *Continuing bonds.* Washington, DC: Taylor & Francis.

Landry-Datteé, Delaigue-Cosset (2001). Support groups for children. *European Journal of Palliative Care* **8**(3):107–10.

Lindemann S (1944). Symptomatology and management of acute grief. *American Journal of Psychiatry* **101**:141–8.

Mansell Pattison E (1997). *The experience of dying.* New Jersey: Prentice Hall.

Monroe B, Oliviere D (ed.) (2003). *Patient participation in palliative care.* Oxford: Oxford University Press.

Oliviere D, Hargreaves R, Monroe B (1998). *Good practices in palliative care.* Aldershot: Ashgate Publishing Ltd.

Schon D (1987). *The reflective practitioner.* San Francisco, CA: Jossey Bass.

Sheldon F (1997). *Psychosocial palliative care.* Cheltenham: Stanley Thornes.

Walsh F (ed.) (1993). *Normal family processes.* New York: Guilford Press.

Walsh F, McGoldrick M (1991). *Living beyond loss; death in the family.* London: Norton & Co.

Walter (1994). *Revival of death.* London: Routledge.

Worden(1991). *Grief counselling and grief therapy.* New York: Springer.

Chapter 10

Working with volunteers to provide bereavement support to children

Christine Pentland

The anxiety in the room is palpable. The nine people who are gathered look as if they are anticipating a visit to the dentist, probably without anaesthetic. The challenge for us is clear; we have forty hours to replace anxiety with confidence, to bring knowledge, to enable the personal growth and reflective learning which will enable these individuals to become SeeSaw Support Workers. SeeSaw is a grief support service for children in Oxfordshire, England. We aim to offer a flexible, bespoke support service to children up to the age of eighteen who have been bereaved of a parent or sibling. This service is delivered by a multi-disciplinary team of three full-time clinical members of staff, an administrator, a fund-raiser and a group of volunteer support workers.

Our support workers are the backbone of SeeSaw. It is the Support Workers who, following careful assessment by the clinical team, will offer the one to one support to children and families which is a key component of the repertoire of support that we offer at SeeSaw. It is my aim in this chapter to consider some of the issues and challenges in using volunteers to provide bereavement support to children and families.

SeeSaw came into being when a group of interested and experienced clinicians were brought together to form a working party by Marylyn Relf and Ann Couldrick who had set up the Adult Bereavement Service at Sir Michael Sobell House, a hospice in the United Kingdom. This group consisted of a Consultant Child Psychiatrist, an Educational Psychologist, and a Senior Practioner with Social Services. A report was commissioned by Sir Michael Sobell House Hospice to look at the support needs of bereaved children in Oxfordshire. The key findings of the report were (Couldrick 1997):

- Preventative care for bereaved children in Oxfordshire is limited

- Teachers, Health Visitors, and other professionals whose work role brings them into contact with bereaved children believed that they have much to offer but lack training and access to information and advice

- Bereaved parents wanted more information, advice and support to help understand and respond to children's needs

- Children may express their feelings in different ways according to their age and circumstance but want their individual needs to be recognized and responded to with sensitivity
- There was strong local support for a new initiative specializing in the care of bereaved children and young people.

This report confirmed the conviction that the needs of bereaved children in Oxfordshire were largely unmet and that there was a need for a dedicated children's bereavement service in Oxfordshire.

Clearly the time was right to move this work forward and to establish a new children's bereavement support service. The working party envisaged that this service would be offering support rather than counselling or therapy, and, based on the successful model of support in the bereavement service at Sir Michael Sobell House, would use volunteers.

Historically, volunteers have played a major role in the provision of adult bereavement support within the field of palliative care. In fact, volunteers are the major providers of bereavement care in the UK (Faulkner 1993). The service at Sir Michael Sobell House was a well-established service using volunteers to offer a direct service to bereaved adults. Relf (2000) sums up the advantages of bereavement support as follows:

- Volunteers demonstrate that grief is a normal response to bereavement. The involvement of volunteers demonstrates that the grieving process is a natural and normal, although undoubtedly painful, response to loss
- They are perceived as less distant or less threatening than professionals
- They have the potential to educate and influence others in the community about loss and bereavement
- They understand and represent the local community in a way that professionals cannot
- Volunteers visit the home which is perceived as being less formal than in an office and volunteers are not restricted to the 'counselling hour'
- Volunteers are flexible and are able to take time to accept a cup of tea, look at flowers planted by the deceased etc. Relf's study (2000) found little evidence that this greater informality was connected with dependency problems
- Volunteers are strangers. This enables clients to tell their stories in the knowledge that their helpers have no preconceived ideas but want to know about the deceased and what the loss means
- Giving the four hours per week as suggested by the bereavement service, dilutes the exposure to suffering and loss and means that volunteers are unlikely to get saturated with grief which, according to Kirchberg et al. (1998) reduces the capacity to respond empathically to situations involving death and bereavement.

By 2000 the original core group of Trustees had secured charitable status and had been joined by others from the world of business and finance, and sufficient funding had been secured to enable the appointment of a staff team. A Director was appointed in June 2003 to set up SeeSaw as an operational service. Because the need was so pressing it was essential to get started as quickly as possible. In order to facilitate this it was decided to recruit volunteers who already had considerable expertise and experience in working with children and could therefore be 'fast-tracked' into a support worker role because of their professional backgrounds. Therefore a team of six Support Workers was recruited consisting of an educational psychologist, a social worker specializing in paediatric mental health, two counsellors, a children's hospice worker, and a community psychiatric nurse.

How SeeSaw developed

From the beginning, SeeSaw had shaped its service in direct response to what children, families, and professionals were telling us that they needed from a bereavement service. The Director conducted a series of interviews with families where the death had occurred between two and three years before. After indicating that confidentiality would be maintained they were given the opportunity to say what they had found helpful and unhelpful about professional intervention around the time of their bereavement. They were also asked what they thought a service like SeeSaw could have offered them. Because of the informal nature of these conversations, and the promise of confidentiality, no notes were taken so no attempt was made to quantify this data but recurrent themes were noted. In addition, a focus group was held consisting of children aged from seven to seventeen. All the children had been bereaved of a parent between twelve and eighteen months previously. The children were very keen to contribute and understood that their help was needed to make SeeSaw an effective service. The children gave us valuable insights into their world and were very clear in their ideas about how they could have been supported if SeeSaw had existed at the time of their bereavement. This process which also included consulting with professionals enabled us to develop a range of services within SeeSaw to meet these stated needs

- Information and resources
- School support
- Work with families before death
- Telephone advice
- One to one and family work
- Training and consultancy
- Support for clergy
- Support groups for parents
- Group work for children
- Fun activities.

It was clear from our on-going conversations with bereaved parents that they want an element of choice and control about the help they receive at the time of their bereavement. We have found that the families need different things from the service at different times. These choices are outlined to them at the time of the first assessment visit, which is an opportunity for the family to say what they need and how they think that their needs might be met. It also enables them to understand that they can access the support that feels right for them. It is important to note that SeeSaw only take referrals directly from families although initial enquiries come via family doctors, teachers, health visitors, etc. This policy of family only referral means that the families who use SeeSaw really want our involvement.

The Harvey family's story illustrates the broad scope of services available at SeeSaw and the way that families are encouraged to be in control of the support they access. The Harvey family contacted us six weeks before Jason Harvey died. In response to requests from families for support before death SeeSaw was able, with the support of Macmillan Cancer Relief, to appoint a further full time worker as part of the clinical team in August 2002. This worker visited the family and supplied them with information and resources. The family required no further input at that time. On the day of Mr Harvey's death the family made contact again wishing to discuss issues around the children (two boys aged seven and nine) seeing the body and attending the funeral. Support was also given to the priest conducting the service about suitable readings and how to involve the children. Mrs Harvey also asked that our school worker make contact with the school to support the boys' teachers. A staffroom meeting was held which led to a request for an inset day training session for the school staff. Following this period of intense involvement the family made no contact for two months. Mrs Harvey then felt that the boys would appreciate the opportunity to talk to a support worker and following a further assessment visit this was arranged. The boys chose to be seen together at home and a volunteer support worker was allocated to the family. Mrs Harvey also accepted an invitation to an informal open access group for parents. The Support Worker visited the family nine times, helping them to preserve their memories and giving them an opportunity to explore their feelings.

It is clear from the story of the Harvey family that SeeSaw is very much focused on offering support and information; we do not call ourselves a counselling service. One of the most important aspects of the service is the normalizing of the bereavement experience and this can sometimes be the only intervention that families need. The assessment visit always includes this element of 'normalizing' and it is a huge relief to families to know that what they are feeing is normal and that the children reactions are as we would expect. We have found that supporting parents is a very effective way of supporting the children and that an early visit to the family which offers this can be all the input that they need. The quality of child-care and the child's relationship with the surviving parent have been consistently identified as key factors that influence the course and outcome of the child's bereavement experience (Brier *et al.* 1988; Worden 1997; Tennant 1998). Therefore, support for parents in the form of an informal parents' group and the opportunity to discuss concerns in individual sessions are offered. Families that do go on to see a support worker understand that we are not offering therapy or counselling although counselling skills are used. The experience of SeeSaw is that our intervention consists of explaining that children need information and reassurance and offering a safe place for the child to explore their feelings of loss and build the memories that they are so fearful of losing.

Volunteers and SeeSaw

It is our conviction that this work of support can be done by specially trained and selected volunteer workers. However, this belief must be bolstered by careful selection procedures, initial and on-going training, and supervision.

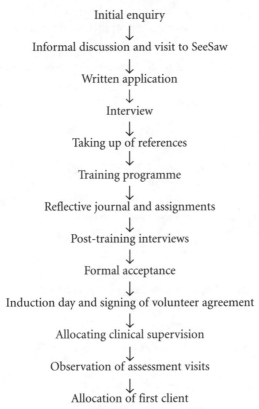

Seesaw Selection Process

Initial enquiry
↓
Informal discussion and visit to SeeSaw
↓
Written application
↓
Interview
↓
Taking up of references
↓
Training programme
↓
Reflective journal and assignments
↓
Post-training interviews
↓
Formal acceptance
↓
Induction day and signing of volunteer agreement
↓
Allocating clinical supervision
↓
Observation of assessment visits
↓
Allocation of first client

Recruiting and appointing new volunteers involves clarity of thinking on the part of the organization about exactly what is wanted from the volunteer. There are the needs of three groups to consider.

- the needs of the organization
- the needs of the clients
- the needs of the volunteer.

The needs of the organization

The organization needs:

- volunteers who show commitment—to training, to the work, to the children, and families

- volunteers who are mentally robust, who can tolerate, and not be frightened by, strong feelings
- volunteers who are willing to reflect on their own loss and who have a belief in the ability of the client to develop inner strength and to grow through the experience of bereavement
- volunteers who are realistically able to fulfil the time commitment
- volunteers who can treat each client as an individual and not be tied to fixed expectations about the duration or frequency of their need for support
- volunteers who have the support of their family and friends
- volunteers who can add value to the service and supplement resources.

The needs of the client

The client needs:

- a worker who is sensitive to their needs
- a support worker who makes a commitment and sticks to it; broken appointments and unpredictability are not helpful
- a worker who can stay with them through difficult emotional experiences without panicking or trying to move them away from difficult feelings
- a worker who can be flexible and who is not tied to their own agenda. 'Yes Johnny, I know you are angry but today we are doing a lovely salt sculpt!'
- a volunteer who is committed to learning about the way that children grieve and how best they can be supported in that grieving process.

The needs of the volunteer

The volunteer needs:

- to feel supported
- to feel a valued part of the team
- opportunities to gain experience and learn new skills
- to be able to identify with the aims and ethos of the organization
- to feel connected with the organization and to feel that they can make a difference and offer a unique contribution that will be celebrated and recognized.

McCurley and Lynch (1994) suggest that organizational climate will influence how volunteers can be involved. Volunteers will quickly become aware of overall attitudes within the organization. The sometimes subtle cues regarding organizational style will influence volunteers' assessment of whether the organization is worth the donation of their time. McCurley and Lynch have identified indicators of a good organizational climate as:

- Clear sense of individual roles, with respect for roles of others
- Willingness to sacrifice for a goal

- Tolerance and acceptance
- Open and honest communication
- Group identity: 'we're in this together'
- Inclusion, not exclusion
- Mutual support and interdependence.

In addition, the organization that welcomes volunteers must be able to show evidence of clear thinking in its procedures, policies, and paperwork in support of a volunteer programme. These include recruitment policies, volunteer management policies, job descriptions, etc. Paperwork needs to be developed to monitor the activity of volunteers such as time sheets and expense forms. Consideration must also be given to Equal Opportunities, Health and Safety and Child Protection procedures. It is good practice for all volunteers to be given a manual containing these policies.

Early on in the history of SeeSaw we advertised for volunteers using posters displayed in a variety of locations such as hospitals and libraries. Interested people were then invited to an Information Evening which gave them an opportunity to find out more about SeeSaw and the commitment required as a Support Worker Volunteer. Approximately 20% of the individuals who attended these information evenings went on to apply to be Support Workers. More recently we have found that we get sufficient numbers of potential volunteers via self-recruitment. They are attracted to the organization, often born of personal or professional experience and have a commitment to the aims and objectives of the service. Others come to us 'by association' because they have a friend who has begun to work for SeeSaw. A small number have come because they wish to gain experience in the field of childhood bereavement with a view to enhancing their future employment prospects.

All potential volunteers are invited to SeeSaw for an informal meeting with the Director. This gives an opportunity for both parties to explore issues around volunteering. At this point potential volunteers are given an information pack with detailed application form, copies of the volunteer agreement, and SeeSaw policies and procedures. If the potential volunteer wishes to proceed with the application they would then fill out the form and nominate two referees.

Interview

The volunteer is interviewed by the Director and one trustee representing the clinical sub group of Trustees. The interview lasts for approx one hour and explores seven key areas:

- relevant qualifications and experience
- motivation and understanding of the role
- recent losses/life events
- reflection/self awareness
- self identified strengths and skills
- self-care and work/life balance

- personal beliefs and values
- transport and availability.

The interview is an opportunity to ensure that the volunteer has a thorough understanding of the role of support worker and is aware of the extent of commitment required. There are three outcomes of the interview:

1. The volunteer is accepted for training; however this does not mean that they will automatically be accepted as a support worker at the end of the training course.
2. The volunteer is offered an alternative role within SeeSaw, e.g. fund-raising.
3. The volunteer is not accepted to work with SeeSaw.

Following acceptance for training, references are taken up and all volunteers are police checked. Police checks are carried out on all volunteers even if their work role requires them to have a current police check. If references and police checks are satisfactory the volunteer is offered a place on the training programme which takes place annually.

Training programme

The SeeSaw training programme consists of a forty-hour training course. In addition to the taught element of the course, volunteers are also required to complete a reflective learning journal and a practical project to design a resource to be used in working with bereaved children. It was felt that the learning experience of the course should reflect the way that we would be working with our clients. Care was taken to foster an atmosphere of trust in which people felt able to share openly. This was important, as the course requires the participants to reflect on their own experience of loss and to share learning and insights with others in the group.

One important early feature of the course is the negotiation of the learning contract in which each participant has the opportunity to say what they need from the group in order to feel safe. Each group writes its own contract but we have noticed that certain key elements are always mentioned. These are the need for security around confidential information, the need for respect for each other's ideas and the need for humour and fun. The contract is developed and each of these themes are explored to ensure that everyone is clear about what is meant by confidentiality, respect, and humour. We have found in the past that these can mean very different things to each participant and consensus and clarity are vital ingredients in enabling people to feel safe within the group.

The use of experiential exercises such as life collages (a craft activity, which identifies significant life experiences), salt sculpts (a creative tool to preserve memories of a person who has died) and geneograms (which explore family relationships) give the volunteers direct knowledge of these powerful interventions. They learn how a child might feel when faced with such exercises and just what support is needed from a helper when completing them. Role-play and Sculpting are used to enable the volunteers not only to practice the role of helper in a safe environment but also to gain insight into family dynamics. It is important always to see the child in context and for the volunteers to appreciate how their work may impact on the child's family and social networks. This blend of theoretical input and practical experience has been well received in evaluations.

The course has been accredited by The Open College Network. The course objectives are:

Personal content

The participants will:

- develop a better understanding of their own experience of loss
- have the opportunity to explore personal anxieties about loss through death
- develop an understanding of loss using their own experience as a baseline.

Theory

The participants will:

- become familiar with the theoretical understanding of bereavement
- understand how a child's developmental stage influences the experience of loss
- understand the context of bereavement support, e.g. family systems, schools, and peer groups.

Practical experience

The participants will:

- develop basic listening and counselling skills based on the work of Rogers (1961) and Egan (1994)
- understand the boundaries of the work and the limits of skills, and also understand when and how to refer on
- develop practical skills to enhance the delivery of bereavement support to both adults and children.

The training takes place over 1 weekend, 2 Saturdays, and 7 evenings. The programme is as shown in Table 10.1.

Upon successful completion of the training programme, volunteers attend an induction evening and are given a post-training interview, after which they are finally accepted as support workers. It is at this point that they are asked to sign the SeeSaw Volunteer Agreement. This lays out the roles and responsibilities for both volunteers and the organization. The agreement is also signed by the Director on behalf of the Trustees of SeeSaw.

The Volunteer Support Worker agrees:

- to offer support to bereaved families enabling them to explore their responses to bereavement
- to give approximately sixteen hours per month to SeeSaw this includes visiting, travelling, report writing, and monthly supervision meetings
- to notify SeeSaw in writing with as much notice as possible of extended leave or resignation

Table 10.1 Training Programme

Weekend	Introduction to child development
	group contract and learning journal
	Life collage
	Introduction to child bereavement
Evening 1	Perspectives on adult grief
Evening 2	Anticipatory grief
Evening 3	Talk by a funeral director
Evening 4	The child at School
Saturday 1	Exploring family dynamics
	Skills practice
	Adolescent workshop
Evening 5	A parent's perspective—talk by a bereaved parent
Evening 6	Skills workshop
Evening 7	Managing endings
Saturday 2	Practical skills

- ◆ to adhere to the principles and policies of SeeSaw
- ◆ to maintain confidentiality within the service
- ◆ to participate in annual appraisals
- ◆ to be willing to participate in the monitoring and evaluation of the service. This includes maintaining records and completing paperwork.

    SeeSaw agrees:

- ◆ to co-ordinate the service
- ◆ to provide induction, training, and adequate information to enable the support worker to meet the responsibilities of the role
- ◆ to provide monthly supervisory support and one-to-one support as necessary
- ◆ to provide support groups and on-going training opportunities
- ◆ to respect the individual needs and circumstances of the support worker
- ◆ to adhere to SeeSaw's principles and procedures
- ◆ to offer an appraisal system
- ◆ to reimburse travel and telephone expenses at a rate set by SeeSaw
- ◆ to follow the SeeSaw complaints procedure for dealing with any complaints made by clients
- ◆ to provide insurance cover and professional indemnity insurance for all support workers when carrying out duties requested by SeeSaw
- ◆ to keep adequate personnel records in order that references can be supplied if required.

After observing visits with a member of the team, the support workers will be allocated their first case and arrangements will be made for their supervision sessions. On the induction evening volunteers are given a file containing SeeSaw policies and procedures and given specific instruction regarding responding to child protection issues. All volunteers are given a summary of the child protection procedure on a credit card sized laminated leaflet. This includes emergency contact numbers for the designated child protection officer. In the case of SeeSaw this is the Director.

We take the personal safety of our volunteers very seriously as they may be working off the SeeSaw premises in schools or in a client's home. We have produced personal safety instructions based on those issued by The Suzy Lamplugh Trust which include all workers informing the office of their appointments and carrying a mobile phone at all times. All SeeSaw staff both paid and unpaid are issued with an identity badge with photograph which clients are advised to ask to see.

All client/worker communication is conducted via the office and workers are advised never to give out their personal phone number.

As soon as a support worker becomes active their name is added to our professional indemnity insurance policy which offers cover for any claims made against the worker in connection with the provision of bereavement support.

We know that in using volunteers we have a responsibility for their safety and the safety of the client group. It is our responsibility following careful assessment of the family situation not to place volunteers with clients at risk of suicide, clients known to be abusing drugs or alcohol, or clients with significant mental health problems. Such cases would be seen by the clinical team at SeeSaw. However, it is vital that, as a support service, we know the limits of the service that we are able to provide and to know when and how to refer on to other more appropriate agencies. The aim of allocation of clients would be that the volunteer would feel they were in a situation that played to their strengths and where they could feel comfortable. In the early days of volunteering, workers are asked to work with families whose needs are assessed as being relatively uncomplicated. At the post-training interview the volunteers are asked which situations they would find especially challenging, which age group of children they feel most comfortable with, and which geographical areas they can cover. We aim to place a new volunteer in a family with a good match to these preferences in order to minimize anxiety.

The first visit is a time of great anxiety. Although the volunteers have had opportunities during training to 'practice' the skills they will need using role play, they are still very concerned about not getting it right or of making a situation worse. The volunteers were asked to identify their fears in an exercise during the training. Typical anxieties were:

- that I might be asked to work in too difficult a situation
- that I might get it 'wrong'
- personal safety
- going to a home to be confronted by an angry or abusive parent
- that I won't be good enough.

In terms of listening to these fears and trying to alleviate them we can certainly reassure volunteers that they will be going to homes where a careful assessment visit has already been done. In addition, we have our safety guidelines in place. The other fears concerning being good enough or making things worse are more difficult to tackle. The experience of our colleagues at Sir Michael Sobell House is that these anxieties will lessen over time. In her study of Sir Michael Sobell House bereavement service Relf (2000) found that her quantitative results supported Parkes' (1981) hypothesis that volunteers take time to develop their skills and confidence. Volunteer interviews at Sir Michael Sobell House revealed that inexperienced volunteers were more anxious about their abilities whereas experienced volunteers were more focused on their client. In the early days of their volunteering workers are much more focused on 'doing' and often go armed with many resources and tools with which to gain a child's attention. As time goes by they are much less likely to need the 'security blanket' of resources and come to the place where they realize that the best resource that they have is themselves.

In listening to the anxieties of new volunteers we have found that it is helpful for them to have the opportunity to speak with an experienced volunteer who can help to reassure them that these fears are normal. It is interesting that the level of anxiety appears to be high in all volunteers regardless of their professional background. Such fears are not restricted to volunteers. For example, counselling diploma students also experience more discomfort when working with situations involving death and bereavement (Kirchberg *et al.* 1998).

Relf's study (2000) suggests that, with support, volunteers are able to manage the emotional pain associated with being open to others, feelings of powerlessness at not being able to make it better (Kalish 1985; Parkes 1986), and the dependency issues highlighted by Faulkner (1993) and Raphael *et al.* (1993). She found little evidence that memories of personal losses (Raphael *et al.* 1993) caused problems for volunteers or that the work was unduly distressing.

At SeeSaw we have found that the key component in the recognition and support and management of such anxiety is the supervisory relationship.

Supervision

Supervision is viewed as an essential and non-negotiable element of the volunteer's commitment. The work of bereavement support is challenging and will have a personal impact. Relf (2000) noted that 'volunteers may identify with their clients, feel helpless or anxious'. Bereavement support is stressful and will awaken past feelings of loss and separation. Supervision is a safe place to explore these and other issues which may arise from the volunteer's work. Thus supervision becomes a vital part of the culture of learning and support that we wish to develop. Supervision also gives space for reflection and the monitoring of standards. Kadushin (1976) identifies the functions of supervision as managerial, educative, and supportive. This has become the three-way model of supervision provided for our volunteers. It also gives opportunity for the monitoring of standards thereby protecting the client. It gives the worker space to reflect on the content and process of their work and to develop understanding and practical skills. Finally, it gives the organization the opportunity to safeguard against burnout. Ignoring the impact of what Raphael *et al.* (1993) call 'the painfulness of empathy' could result in volunteers resigning because the work becomes too stressful for them. In terms of volunteer support it appears to be better to build a fence at the top of the cliff than put an ambulance at the bottom. Supervision is that fence. It is the safety feature of volunteer management that helps to prevent the loss of volunteers through burnout.

In the mid-1980s the National Council for Voluntary Organizations (undated document) produced guidelines for setting up a bereavement project. Here, it was suggested that volunteers should be provided with a monthly support group of 1½ hours led by an experienced person and that up to eight volunteers could be supervised in this way. Again drawing on the experience of the bereavement service at Sir Michael Sobell House we felt that this was not sufficient for our workers. Following the Sobell model we decided to offer a combination of small and large group supervision. To offer individual supervision on a monthly basis proved to be too costly and time consuming so the volunteers were allocated to groups of two or three people. Each group is led by an experienced practitioner and 1½ hours are set aside for each group. Supervisors meet quarterly with the Director to discuss issues of concern and clinical governance.

We also offered monthly group meetings. Initially we struggled to find the right format for this group. We were suffering because we were trying our best to meet everyone's needs. Some were asking for further training, some wanted open case discussion, some wanted a more formal case presentation, others wanted to develop skills, and some others were clearly looking for a more social evening. The group contract that has now evolved incorporates an element of most of these.

The need for the volunteers to meet each other as a whole group cannot be underestimated. This fosters the group identity and goes some way in combating the feelings of isolation that most volunteers tell us that they experience. In addition to the group meetings we have tried to have two social events per year for the team. We want the volunteers to hear the message that they are valued and that they are an essential part of the service. However, it must be acknowledged that we are asking people to work in isolation. This can be a problem as visits are done after office hours so the volunteers do not have access to the staff team if they have had a particularly difficult visit and needed to offload. To combat this, volunteers have been given a mobile number, which they can use in these circumstances. Whilst all the volunteers appreciated this and felt that it would be helpful it is rarely used.

Part of the supervision process is the annual appraisal system for volunteers. This gives the volunteer the opportunity to review their work for SeeSaw and to identify needs which they might feel are not being met, for example, training requests. The volunteers are asked to complete a self-assessment form before coming for an appraisal interview with two members of the SeeSaw staff team. Volunteers are asked to reflect on their personal goals and objectives for their SeeSaw work and whether these goals have been achieved. They are asked to identify the areas of the work that they find particularly challenging and those that give them the most rewards. They are encouraged to identify ways in which SeeSaw could improve in the organization and support of the volunteers and to look at future training needs. These annual appraisals have given volunteers the opportunity to have a voice in the shaping of the service and will influence future policy and practice.

By reading the annual appraisal forms we have been able to understand the volunteer and their needs more clearly. The volunteers have been able to flag up issues that have been important and this has given us insight into the reasons people volunteer and the support they require to continue in the role.

When asked what they had valued most about their involvement with SeeSaw, the volunteers shared their positive feelings about volunteering:

- the moment when a child gives insight into their feelings
- seeing the children develop skills which are transferable into other areas of their lives
- when a child looks better
- working to increase a parent's understanding of and confidence with their children
- making a difference
- helping to support the whole family
- knowing that I have completed a good piece of work
- seeing positive change
- friendships with other team members
- great training opportunities
- being part of a growing, organic organization
- supportive supervision.

Aspects of the work that volunteers felt to be, more difficult included:

- visiting children at a time when my own children need me at home
- not knowing if I am really helping
- maintaining boundaries between the needs of adults and children
- knowing that in some families adults may not be supportive of the work
- meeting the needs of different age groups when working with a family group
- going home to an empty house after a difficult session
- managing my own feelings
- working in the child's home
- endings.

It would seem from reading these comments that the rewards and pressures of volunteering are very similar to those identified by paid workers. Indeed, the principles of effective volunteer management are much the same as those for good practice in personnel management.

Who volunteers?

A recent study (Rolls and Payne 2003) looked at the provision of children's bereavement services throughout the UK. This included a section on staffing. The study found that of the services included in the study 73% relied on a mixture of paid and unpaid staff, 14% relied entirely on unpaid workers and only 11% relied entirely on paid staff.

Table 10.2 SeeSaw Support Workers July 2003

Child psychotherapists	2
Counsellors	4
Education	6
Psychologist	1
Other	1

The study found that whether paid or unpaid, services were staffed by a significant number of people with professional qualifications. The use of the term 'volunteer' has often been associated with 'amateur' or 'unqualified' (which is one of the reasons we call our volunteers support workers) but within SeeSaw the majority of our volunteers have a relevant professional qualification (Table 10.2).

The average age for SeeSaw volunteers is forty-seven. We have only one male volunteer and have had very little interest from men wishing to volunteer. We have had five enquiries from men about becoming support workers but only one of these progressed to interview. About 50% of our volunteers are in full-time employment, 25% work part-time and the remaining 25% work in the home or are retired.

Retention issues

Since January 2000 SeeSaw has trained a total of twenty-four people for the role of volunteer support worker. By September 2003 a total of fourteen were still active as support workers, four people have resigned as support workers and the remaining six have asked for a leave of absence (Table 10.3).

The six support workers who have asked for a leave of absence (provision for which is written into our volunteer agreement) have all cited family commitments as the reason for their request. All of these volunteers have school age children. All of them have asked for leave of absence within twelve months of joining SeeSaw and have all had only three clients or less. Of the support workers who have been active for more than twelve months, none have young children. This has led us to the conclusion that being a support worker may not be compatible with a young family. There may be several reasons for this:

- SeeSaw offers families the choice about when they will be seen. Most families choose the gap between school and teatime. This means that support workers with young families are likely to be asked to work at the very time when needed by their own family.

Table 10.3 Reasons for resigning

Pregnancy	1
Ill health	1
Further study	1
Unable to cope with the work	1

- SeeSaw workers are using arts and crafts to help the children, as one volunteer said 'I was doing things with other people's children that I never make time to do with my own'
- Although asked at interview about the support that will be available from a spouse this is often a source of tension as a spouse left at home with small children can become resentful
- Volunteers found that their own children were unhappy about them going out to see other children
- Issues of transference could become more difficult when dealing with children the same age as your own.

These facts have led us to be much more rigorous in outlining the possible difficulties for parents of young children at interview. Potential volunteers who have young families are made aware of the difficulties that others have reported so we know that they are making an informed choice about volunteering and are realistic about the commitment involved.

Conclusions

One of the myths surrounding the use of volunteers in services such as SeeSaw is that it is a cheap option. I would like to explode that myth here and now. Volunteer workers may be cost effective but they are not free of cost. The costs involved are:

- recruitment
- administration of applications
- police checks—in some areas there may be a charge for this although SeeSaw has been able to negotiate free police checks
- training—venue, resources, tutor time, refreshments
- administration of volunteer activity
- professional indemnity insurance
- supervision—this has proved one of the most costly aspects of volunteer related activity
- support by staff team—This cannot be underestimated. Volunteers are given 'carte blanche' to contact the office whenever they need support. Especially in the early days of their volunteering, support workers make frequent contact with the office. This can be demanding in an already overstreched team
- travel and other expenses
- on-going training
- social events.

Relf's research (2000) demonstrated that volunteers can work in partnership with professionals to provide a bereavement service. She considers such services sustainable depending on the availability of funding, the infrastructure available to support them and on maintaining positive views about volunteers. Despite the high degree of commitment required, the demanding nature of the work and the impact of women's increased participation in paid employment, the service at Sir Michael Sobell House has continued to develop and to attract new volunteers. Certainly we have found that at SeeSaw we have many people interested in volunteering and already have a waiting list for the next training session. The temptation would be to increase the volunteer team numbers but experience has taught us that a team of more than sixteen volunteers presents logistical problems that are difficult to manage. The most significant issue when the numbers exceeded sixteen was that the quality individual support and personal interest in the progress of each volunteer was diluted to the point where volunteers started to report that they felt out of touch with the organization.

A study of the use of volunteers to provide bereavement support to children and families would be interesting and fruitful. Relf (2000) describes volunteer bereavement support as 'the relatively uncharted territory between traditional concepts of volunteer and professional roles.' There is certainly a need for more work to evaluate the effectiveness of using volunteers to provide bereavement support to children. A further interesting area for research would explore why the majority of volunteers in the world of children's bereavement services are female and tend to be over forty. As a service less than four years old SeeSaw has not yet been able to look at these issues in any depth. Our evidence is largely anecdotal, based on conversations with volunteers and the more formal annual appraisal documents.

However, we do know and gratefully acknowledge that at SeeSaw we would be providing a significantly reduced service if we did not use our unpaid workers.

We know how much we owe to our support workers who give so freely of themselves to share the journey through grief with the children and families. They are often told 'I don't know how you could do this work' and then when people find out that they are not being paid they are even more incredulous. To watch children and adults growing through the experience of loss is reward enough anchored in the belief that people can get through the acute pain of bereavement with the right support from others. As Archbishop Anthony Bloom said in The David Kissen Memorial lecture in 1969.

> People are much greater and stronger than we imagine, and when the unexpected tragedy comes ... we see them grow to a stature that is far beyond anything we imagined. We must remember that people are capable of greatness, of courage, but not in isolation ... They need the conditions of a solidly linked human unit, in which everyone is prepared to bear the burdens of others.

References

Brier A, Kelso J, Kirwin P, et al. (1988). Early parental loss and development of adult psychopathology. *Archives of General Psychiatry* **45**:987–93.

Couldrick A (1997). The support needs of bereaved children and young people in Oxfordshire. Unpublished research report. Oxford: Sir Michael Sobell House.

Egan (1994). *The Skilled Helper.* California: Brookes-Cole.

Faulkner A (1993). Developments in bereavement services. In: D Clark (ed.) *The future for palliative care: issues of policy and practice.* Buckingham: Open University Press.

Kadushin A (1976). *Supervision in social work.* New York: Columbia University Press.

Kalish RA (1985). *Death, grief and the caring relationship*, 2nd edn. California: Brooks Cole.

Kaplan AG (ed.) (1983). *Work in progress 2: women and empathy.* Wellesley College, MA: Stone Centre for Developmental Services and Studies.

Kirchberg TM, Niemayer RA, James RK (1998). Beginning counsellors' death concerns and empathic responses to clients' situations involving death and grief. *Death Studies* 22:99–120.

McCurley S, Lynch R (1994). *Essential volunteer management.* London: DCS.

Parkes CM (1986). *Counselling in terminal care and bereavement.* Leicester: British Psychological Society Books.

Raphael B, Middleton W, Martinek N, Misso V (1993). Counselling and therapy of the bereaved. In: MS Stroebe, W Stroebe, RO Hansson (ed.) *Handbook of bereavement.* Cambridge: Cambridge University Press.

Relf M (2000). *The effectiveness of volunteer bereavement care. An evaluation of a palliative care bereavement service.* Unpublished PhD Thesis, University of London.

Rogers CR (1961). *On becoming a person.* London: Constable.

Rolls L, Payne S (2003). Childhood bereavement services: a survey of UK provision. *Palliative Medicine* 17:423–32.

Tennant C (1988). Parental loss in childhood: its effect in adult life. *Archives of General Psychiatry* 45:1045–9.

Worden W (1997). *Children and grief–when a parent dies.* New York: Guilford Press.

Chapter 11

Loss and grief in school communities[1]

Louise Rowling

Introduction

Over the past decade or so, global terrorism and violence have become part of the everyday lives of individuals, communities, and nation states, not only because of the exposure given to events by the global media coverage, but also due to the targeting of previously 'safe' environments such as: workplaces, social gatherings in clubs and hotels, and schools. A critical point in terms of potential impact on people in this exposure is the intimacy in the reporting of these tragic events. It is these events and their reporting that has contributed to experiences of loss, either real or vicarious, becoming as in times past, a more mainstream part of life in Western communities. That is, these events and experiences are ceasing to be seen as private individual or family matters. In this context the need for dual processes of community recovery and individual and family support becomes imperative.

Reconceptualizing grief as a globalized as well as local personal phenomenon provides the opportunity to move it from an individualized pathologized experience, the purview of the counselling profession, to a 'normal' life event where restorative community processes provide support (Rowling 2003). Viewed from this perspective loss can be placed not only in a psychological framework with concomitant individual and group support processes, but within the aegis of public health and social institutions such as faith communities and schools. To effectively support young people through schools, approaches and processes are needed that are based on the recognition of a wider framework for grief experiences. This wider framing facilitates understanding the impact these events have on school community members when the sense of safety, trust, and predictability of life for people in the environments of their everyday lives is disrupted. Validating, restorative, and enfranchizing approaches need to be created

---

[1]Many of the ideas in this chapter are delineated in greater details in Rowling, L (2003) *Grief in school communities: effective support strategies*, Buckingham, Open University Press

in school communities. A reorientation of practices of service providers may be needed in short term interventions within this framework.

The frameworks of public health, in particular, mental health promotion and prevention, and the health promoting school (healthy schools) underpin this chapter. They are used as models for a multi-level approach where individuals and their social worlds are identified as important. Within this perspective, suggestions for action are identified.

Individual in the context of their school community

Individuals and groups have been the focus of much of the research and interventions in the field of thanatology. The immediate needs individuals present are undoubtedly a powerful basis for theorizing, research, and for developing effective interventions. But for children and young people, by concentrating on an individual's experience divorced from its context, we have failed to embed their issues of concern in a social environment. For most young people, after the family this context involves the school and its community. By isolating grief as a phenomenon we have also failed to locate it in the wider health field. Additionally the focus has often been too much on the pathology of grief. It could be argued that this focus has been necessary to establish grief as a legitimate area through comprehensive research and practice. But it is time to re-conceptualize the area, from a concentration on individuals' experiences to an equal place in the research and practice for the contextual variables within which the bereavement occurs. This reorientation of the field involves placing loss and grief, as a normal life experience, within the mental health promotion field, not within an illness individually centred framework. This ideological shift will broaden the scope for interventions. It is based on the focus of the last decade or two of the need to see loss experiences as interpreted through social interaction (Averill and Nunley 1988). This chapter examines the role of the school as a social institution. In this environment young people look to peers and teachers in their schools to:

◆ help define the reality of their losses;

◆ express feelings associated with them;

◆ provide support and access to information; and

◆ help integrate the experience into their lives (Rowling 2003).

The school is not only a social institution for young people, it is also a workplace for staff, all of whom spend many hours there. It can provide an environment (in terms of policies, programs, and practices) that is supportive as well as access to individuals who can provide help through formal and informal mechanisms.

Loss and grief as a mental health issue in schools, embeds experiences in the wider field of school health. Current global evidence in school health no longer concentrates on the curriculum as the sole focus for bringing about health behaviour change in schools. The comprehensive approach to school health embodied in the health promoting schools framework or healthy schools, acknowledges the wider impact of the psychosocial environment in the school as well as the contribution of family and community. The three areas of action that comprise the health promoting schools framework are: curriculum, teaching, and learning; school organization, ethos, and environment; and partnerships and services (Fig. 11.1). Addressing loss and grief in schools by action in each of these areas creates a supportive context.

Health promoting schools also accomplish more than addressing health issues in schools in a comprehensive way—such as creating policy to support curriculum or changing the physical environment to make the healthy choices the easy choices. It involves providing conditions for the empowerment of the school community to take ownership of the health of its community, thereby being proactive for health issues the community has identified, rather than being reactive to the agendas of outside bodies. This approach has significant implications for short-term bereavement interventions for grieving students or if a critical incident occurs in a school.

For this comprehensive approach to support and enhance short term interventions, service providers may need to shift their work practices from a sole focus on crisis intervention to include proactive partnerships with school communities. This will involve actively working with school personnel to tailor support to meet their expressed needs. It may require changes in roles from grief experts to facilitators and supporters of school staff actions. Conceptualizing loss and grief within the social environment of the school is a theoretically and practically sound strategy. It acknowledges the role of the school organizational factors that can facilitate the creation of a context that accepts the 'normality of grief'. This is in contrast to a crisis orientated approach which may fail to recognize the school as a community, a social system, which has the capacity to provide support (Petersen and Straub 1992). Within this social system there can be norms and rules that sanction or block young people's experience of grief (Rowling 1999).

A validating community

The emphasis in this chapter is on building the capacity of the school community to achieve a comprehensive approach to the grief experiences of its members. Silverman and Worden (1992) identified that following the death of a parent, children who received support at home and in school displayed fewer behavioural problems, than those who did not have similar support networks. The loss experiences of teachers and students can be validated through curriculum, pastoral care processes, critical incident management plans and policies, and special leave policies for staff.

Using a framework for mental health promotion and prevention in schools (Fig. 11.2) delineates levels of intervention and provides a system of care within an environment that acknowledges the varying needs that exist in a school community (Sheehan et al. 2002). This framework can be used to develop a comprehensive approach to loss and grief (Fig. 11.3).

It is important within a comprehensive framework that particular processes and practices are used to connect these levels of care. Whilst diagrammatically they are separated they need to be viewed as seamless levels. Consultation is a vital component in developing a comprehensive approach to grief. Building on existing activities, identifying gaps, and planning school determined procedures are elements of exemplary

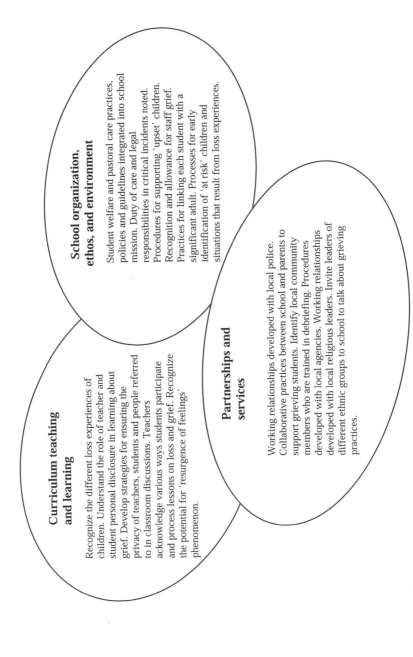

Fig. 11.1 Loss and grief in the health promoting school framework (Rowling 2003).

Curriculum teaching and learning

Recognize the different loss experiences of children. Understand the role of teacher and student personal disclosure in learning about grief. Develop strategies for ensuring the privacy of teachers, students and people referred to in classroom discussions. Teachers acknowledge various ways students participate and process lessons on loss and grief. Recognize the potential for 'resurgence of feelings' phenomenon.

School organization, ethos, and environment

Student welfare and pastoral care practices, policies and guidelines integrated into school mission. Duty of care and legal responsibilities in critical incidents noted. Procedures for supporting 'upset' children. Recognition and allowance for staff grief. Practices for linking each student with a significant adult. Processes for early identification of 'at risk' children and situations that result from loss experiences.

Partnerships and services

Working relationships developed with local police. Collaborative practices between school and parents to support grieving students. Identify local community members who are trained in debriefing. Procedures developed with local agencies. Working relationships developed with local religious leaders. Invite leaders of different ethnic groups to school to talk about grieving practices.

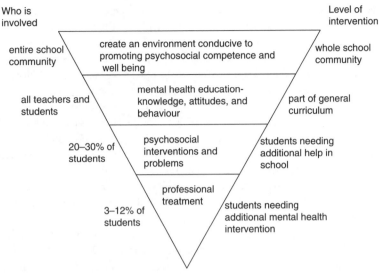

Fig. 11.2 World Health Organization model of school-based mental health promotion.

practice. Members of the community need to experience the synergistic interaction between curriculum, practices, policies, and partnerships with parents and outside providers creating a community of care that validates grief experiences.

School organization, ethos, and environment

Whilst implementing curricula for students about grief or conducting a grief support group are often used as the main preventive activities by outside service providers,

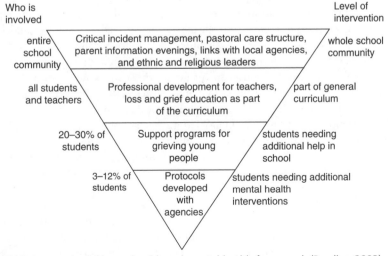

Fig. 11.3 Loss and grief in a school-based mental health framework (Rowling 2003).

these need to be embedded in a wider whole school system of care. This holistic approach to loss and grief involves the hidden curriculum or the ethos of the school. Identifying this is not easy. The ethos of a supportive context includes: the school policies that provide for the emotional welfare of students; a well developed pastoral care system; clear procedures for referral of students to outside agencies; availability of a school-based counselling service; and/or a grief support program. The ethos involves staff relationships—how the school cares for its staff; recognition of the importance of maintaining staff morale; and the relationships between the Head Teacher and individual staff members. Being part of the 'hidden curriculum', school ethos and the attendant belief system that is the basis of a supportive environment, may need to be made explicit. Statements from school leaders that represent the underlying beliefs and philosophies of school practices and policies are one way of achieving this explicitness.

Sensitive issues such as loss and grief create debate and disagreement in school communities. This is due to their characteristics of emotionality, values, beliefs, and past experience combined with the varying perspectives of school community members (Rowling 1996). A school's concern about students' personal well being will be evident in implementation of policies for handling sensitive issues. For example, a critical incident management plan (Yule and Gold 1993) demonstrates a school's commitment to the well being of school community members if a traumatic incident occurs. It is a demonstration of a school's caring ethos. Similarly, inclusive practices can acknowledge varying mourning rituals of different faith communities. Additionally, clear guidelines can be in operation to handle confidentiality and privacy issues for young people. Less obvious policies include assessment policies, where the impact of grief for adolescents that may affect their school performance should be noted. This impact may be immediate, but it can also be delayed, affecting schoolwork months after the loss.

Partnerships and services

The second area of the health promoting school concerns the development of partnerships. These partnerships are with parents as well as outside agencies. Well developed partnerships with outside agencies provide the school with ready access to personnel for referral of 'at risk' students or staff traumatized by violence or other critical incidents. These relationships also provide resources that can assist in educating families, who can then be more supportive and understanding of the experience of their grieving children and siblings. Similarly, partnerships with ethnic and religious leaders bring opportunities for the school to work with these community leaders for support of families.

Small groups with trained facilitators from bereavement support services can provide short-term interventions either on the school grounds and in school time or outside school hours. These support programmes can be helpful for children (Smith and Pennells 1995). But there is also a real need for dialogue with young people—what do they see as helpful? How do they experience events? Dialogue also needs to be encouraged about young people, between service providers and school personnel. Whilst some school personnel and service providers may worry this would jeopardize confidentiality, protocols that elaborate confidentiality versus privacy can help overcome this fear. In this way young people who participate in short-term interventions can be supported in the longer term by school personnel as they adjust to their loss.

In a caring community that validates grief experiences, a very real concern for teachers is—how to respond to an upset child. Setting up procedures to manage such occurrences needs to be done as part of the whole school approach and especially before lessons are taught.

Students become upset in classrooms from time to time, and in discussions about grief the possibility of upset is very real. Useful strategies for supporting upset students inside and outside the classroom include (Rowling 2003):

- choosing a private moment to ask them if they're OK
- avoiding directing attention towards that student
- giving them space within the classroom to be upset
- offering them a chance to leave the room and get a drink/tissue and to return when more composed
- allowing them to go to some designated quiet place in the school or to a predetermined person such as a nurse or counsellor
- offering a buddy to accompany them if immediate comfort is needed
- following up with the student after the event or lesson
- setting a task for other students while you sit and talk with the upset student.

Curriculum

Within a mental health promotion framework loss experiences are part of a curriculum that is proactive in that it is not developed after a crisis but included as a part of existing personal, social, and life skills programmes. This is a natural way to incorporate exploration of feelings of grief and experiences associated with loss. This approach facilitates the normalization of grief through education (Zisook 1987). Mental preparation and planning before a death or other critical event occurs, leads to a much better handling than if one 'takes things as they come'. The orientation of curriculum would not just involve understanding feelings of loss and reactions as in past curriculum approaches, but would include the teaching of skills, to enable individuals to cope and/or to be supportive to others (Glassock and Rowling 1991).

Educating young people about grief is not just about 'feelings' there are competencies and life skills that need to be developed. These are (Rowling 2003):

- knowledge about loss and grief reactions;
- skills to use the information to help themselves;
- knowledge and skills to seek help and recognize when support would be beneficial;
- how to use information about loss experiences to understand and support others; and
- how the knowledge and skills about loss and grief assist them to be a supportive school community member and so the feeling of 'difference' a grieving young person may experience is minimized.

Training for teachers to teach about loss and grief and the active learning styles utilized, is necessary. The sensitivity in the teaching is a result of the personal experiences of teachers, the pedagogy, as well as the content. There are professional challenges for teachers in responding to students who get upset when they disclose emotional life events that are triggered by the lesson. In these instances teacher needs to develop expertise in balancing the aims of the lessons with creating an open and trusting environment where students feel comfortable to share their experiences. Keeping this balance is a formidable task for teachers especially when approaching these lessons for the first time. But as one senior student affirmed it was important:

> It's not going to do you any good if you've got a wonderful mark in maths if your personal life is totally ruined, because you did not deal with a problem properly. It's balance, a well rounded education (Nicole, 16-year-old student).[2]

Students respond positively to teachers who are prepared to devote time to issues that impact on their lives, issues that families and some communities can treat as taboo topics. The result of taboos is that many young people still grieve silently and alone. School education is needed to increase acceptance by a young person's peers of the impact of loss. To achieve this, children and adolescents need to be taught about loss and grief as a normal part of their education, so that they can understand their own experiences and limit the sanctions that they apply to their peers.

Allan reported that he felt his friends understood his situation. His mother was very ill. She had frequent life threatening fits that often required immediate treatment. He needed to be at home in the evening in case his mother needed help. He had accepted this and so had his friends:

> Most of my friends understand. They ask me to sleep over and I say 'No'. They know I have a good reason for staying home and looking after Mum.
>
> (Allan, 14 years old)

Teachers may feel ill equipped to manage loss issues and view this role as one more thing they are being asked to do. They may see themselves as a teacher of a subject and in comparison to bereavement service providers, that they lack expert knowledge that they perceive as needed to manage grief issues. Nevertheless they are concerned about issues that impact on children's academic achievement. A child's school work is likely to be affected by bereavement (Corr and Balk 1999). Teachers can support grieving families by alerting them to any changes of behaviour in their children in school.

Service providers have a significant role to play in providing technical support to teachers and modelling effective teaching pedagogy. This may involve being open to hearing young people's experiences, providing answers to questions frequently asked (viz. what happens when you die?), and team teaching to increase a teacher's confidence and comfort level. A support team to staff teaching in the area is necessary to defuse issues that might arise for the teacher, for example a teacher feeling guilty if students become distressed in the classroom as a result of the lesson.

---

[2]In this chapter verbatim anonymized quotations are used from research more fully reported in Rowling (2003).

Training is necessary for teachers to (Rowling 2003):

♦ develop good communication skills;

♦ be aware of grief and bereavement patterns;

♦ identify their feelings about their own loss experiences;

♦ know the content and process of grief education;

♦ be aware of school policies and procedures about critical incident management;

♦ know how to support an upset child;

♦ maintain links with service providers; and

♦ accept loss and grief as part of life.

With this training teachers can be supportive to families particularly to those who are isolated in the community. This can be achieved by:

♦ practical advice about how to explain death to a child and answer their questions;

♦ acting as the link to agencies and services; and

♦ participating in mourning rituals at the family's request.

In this way a sense of belonging and connection to the school community can be created. This can facilitate natural recovery processes for the family.

The technical expertise of bereavement agencies needs to be employed to support school communities in their efforts to address loss and grief. Unless this happens children's grief will continue to be handled ineffectively. It will still be seen as 'abnormal' and therefore the job of psychologists or social workers. Those in support roles to schools may need to determine what quality practice entails in this area. By embedding loss and grief in the wider issues of concern of teachers such as behaviour problems or general emotional adjustment, the possibility of teachers taking an interest in the area is increased. That is, linking young people's grief experiences to issues teachers are already concerned about creates a possibility that loss and grief will be taken up as a legitimate responsibility for school communities.

Linking loss and grief into the wider picture of mental health in schools helps to counter resistance from school personnel. It does not ask them to be social workers, but locates their current practice in a hierarchy of interventions (Figure 11.3), where there is a clear role identified for them and the potential contribution of specialized helpers is indicated.

Despite the personal and professional challenges those teachers who do acknowledge grief in their students' lives, believe that teaching all students about grief as a life experience and supporting grieving young people is part of their role as a teacher. They see it as relating to students so that they feel confident in the learning situation, a necessary state if they are to achieve their educational goals (Rowling 2003).

The school/community interface includes interagency collaboration for referral for health problems such as staff traumatized by violence from students; and inclusion of outside agencies such as the police and community health centre in the planning and delivery of policies and programmes such as critical incident management. It also includes parent/school liaison in curriculum consultation about loss and grief; critical incident management plan implementation; and teacher/parent communication about grieving adolescents. Another aspect of the community outreach could be education for family and friends. This education could be provided through the school by an outside agency. It has been advocated as a way to help families accept the expression of feelings, gain insight into their own grief, and help them support other family members (Zisook 1987).

The comprehensive approach described in this chapter will help create a supportive environment. In this environment, enfranchisement of those whose grief is not recognized can occur (see description later in this chapter).

A restorative community

After short-term interventions, a longer term need is for restoration. School communities can create environments that support young people. This is one restorative process but there is an additional need in schools when the loss is a result of violence invading not only individuals' lives, but also affecting the geographic space and the social environment of the school. In the latter instance, a violation of the sense of safety of the school may be experienced. The feelings of safety in the school environment need to be recreated, the school being reclaimed as an environment where order, structure, and predictability facilitate the daily routines of teaching and learning. Reclaiming rituals allow for feelings to be collectively constructed and expressed through actions. They create a space, a structure with boundaries where school community members can feel safe to express their tears or reflect on their inner sadness. It is also a place where a sense of hope and faith in the future can be initiated. School leaders can provide guidance for the community response, especially where there is confusion, anger, and doubt. For example Matt, a headteacher described the feeling he had when he walked into his school grounds after a young man unconnected to the school had hanged himself in the playground:

> They [the school community] felt very, very intruded upon. And the gravity of having someone commit suicide where you spend a lot of your time pumping emotional energy into, it is very, very difficult. Adults had to reclaim the place for the kids and that was my role to start the process of reclaiming the place for the school community (Matt, headteacher for 17 years).

Similarly in another school, a student was murdered on the way home from school along a familiar shortcut frequented by many students. The students with the help of the local government public works department and the wider community cleared the track of vegetation and lighting was installed. A formal pathway was declared for the school and the students organized a dedication ceremony. It was through this collective action that the students expressed their grief and reclaimed the violated space. Teachers who bring parents and families into these restorative activities allowing contact and engagement with their child's peers, can facilitate the recovery process for the family. The memories of connectedness and safety generated by rituals created by students and other school community members can provide reassurance long after the ceremonies have occurred.

An enfranchising community

The outcome for staff and students where their school community is not validating and restorative is that they can be disenfranchised grievers. Disenfranchised grief is defined as: 'the grief that persons experience when they incur a loss that is not or cannot be openly acknowledged, publicly mourned, or socially supported'. (Doka 1989, p. 4)

There are five triggers for disenfranchised grief:

◆ The relationship is not recognized;

◆ The loss is not recognized;

◆ Society does not give the person that role (Doka 1989)

◆ The circumstances of the loss;

◆ The ways individuals grieve (Doka 2002).

There are a number of sources of disenfranchised grief in a school community—self, others, and the social world of the school. Whilst there are similarities between schools, each school is unique with their own history, relationships, rules, and procedures that often reflect particular cultural and religious values, beliefs, and normative behaviour. This is especially important because meanings about loss experiences (cognitive representations of reality) come from the culture and others' expectations mediated through an individual's internal resources and life experience (Rowling 2002).

For young people there are different ways their grief is disenfranchised. These can be intrapersonal, interpersonal, or environmental. Intrapersonal sources include fear of social disapproval; fear of loss of control linked to their emerging independence; and the current perceptions and interpretations of their world. Young males in particular are subject to disenfranchisement due to the varying ways they process grief (Martin and Doka 2000). For them psychoeducation, information giving about the normality of grief; classroom discussions about loss and grief; and the 'hearing of others' stories' provides a structure for their thinking, a way to process their grief. It is important to recognize that young men may not talk about their experiences and feelings, but they can still be processing and organizing their thoughts, as Ricardo described:

> It is good to hear about what others are saying. You can just sit there and listen and you have a conversation with yourself, in your mind, you turn it over and that helps. It gives you ideas about how you might explain yourself if you were in that situation.
>
> (Rowling 2002)

What is needed is school environments that validate the varying ways of expressing grief, sanctioning options for young males of diversion and reflection (Martin and Doka 2000), processing by action rather than verbally expressing feeling and by thinking it through rather than talking.

For young people, two sources of interpersonal disenfranchisement are parents and peers. Peer relationships exemplify the paradox of disenfranchised grief. Peers can provide support by words and action, but these mechanisms also do the disenfranchising. To address this, education needs to occur with peers concurrently with provision of support to the griever. Parents and teachers also underestimate the extent of young people's reactions to disasters (Pfefferbaum *et al.* 1999). Reporting a study of youth after the Oklahoma City bombing Pfefferbaum encourages 'active inquiry about symptoms of trauma and grief', because it can be hidden by young people (Rowling 2002). The chronically ill and/or dying adolescent is especially vulnerable to adult sanctions. Adults may deny them the opportunity to take risks as part of their developing independence (Rowling 2002). As part of their anticipatory grief they may not be given the space to discuss the 'what ifs', thereby working towards a cognitive understanding of the certainty of death (Stevens and Dunsmore 1996).

The third source of disenfranchisement is their environment, the organizational rules about grieving and the wider community practices about responding to losses. The extra threat posed by society's attitudes to young people who are already vulnerable because of a loss experience and developmental challenges, creates a triple burden (Rowling 2002). Additionally adults may believe it is not the school's role to be proactive in creating a school environment, where grief is normal and grieving acceptable (Rowling 1999; Rowling and Holland 2000). School environments that sanction grief would acknowledge the loss experiences of young people; support them individually and in groups, and have plans in place to manage critical incidents involving death and loss (Rowling 2002).

Teachers can be especially supportive of a 'well' sibling when their brother or sister is chronically ill or has died. The grief of these siblings can be disenfranchised by the family environment where, as the 'well' child, their needs may be missed. Teachers can be the 'outsider' to this environment, a supportive adult that the sibling can talk to.

Mental health professionals, bereavement counsellors, and educational psychologists in supporting young people experiencing disenfranchised grief need to ask 'What does the griever need to do? What changes are needed in the social environment, from adults, peers, family members, helping professionals, and the wider community?' There needs to be recognition of the different pathways that young people follow as they learn to cope. Consequently, different interventions will be required for different styles of grieving and different circumstances. Working with individuals will not address the behaviour of their peers towards their loss nor the organizational practices that disenfranchise school community members (Rowling 2002).

Teachers as disenfranchised grievers

Research conducted about 10 years ago identified teachers as disenfranchised grievers (Rowling 1995). This influences their capacity to be supportive. Teaching is a profession where emotional connections are made, it is based on human interactions. Teachers care for their pupils. There exists the belief amongst teachers that you have to hide your emotions to manage a class, when a death occurs. For teachers, there is a real fear of 'breaking down in front of the class'. If something traumatic occurs it is likely to involve intense emotions, often emotions that teachers themselves may not recognize. Being affected by grief and therefore not being able to perform their teaching role, influences a teacher's view of themselves as a competent professional because of the need to feel in control of the situation and to rise above natural emotional responses.

If teachers feel they have let their students down, it affects their worklife in the future and the well being of young people in their care. Uniquely for the teaching profession their grief can be disenfranchised by this personal professional conflict created by their:

◆ need to maintain their humanity as part of their teaching role;

◆ professional beliefs about what behaviour is appropriate; and

◆ duty of care for young people.

Grief creates a role conflict, within which 'control' and 'being human' are key concerns. When the loss is viewed as a 'professional loss', directly related to the work environment, such as the death of a student, colleague or a major accident or public crisis involving school personnel or property, from an organizational perspective, it is essential to create a supportive workplace for all school personnel.

For both teachers and students a critical incident can trigger a resurgence of feelings:

> when feelings related to loss, which can sometimes be unresolved, are triggered by current experiences. They may appear to others to be out of place in relation to the current experience. It is often an unconscious process (Rowling 2003).

In the management of an incident in a school there needs to be recognition of the existence of earlier events, particularly those that have occurred in the school with their potential to revive memories. Support, the social sanctioning of grief, needs to be embedded in the school's normal processes. The sanctioning of grief reactions to a crisis provides an opportunity 'for a grief that was disenfranchised many years earlier to emerge and be acknowledged' (Kauffman 1989).

Whilst the needs of staff have been mentioned in texts about school management of crises (Petersen and Straub 1992) most attention in these texts is focussed on the needs of students. A sentence in a British text acknowledges that staff often have a desperate need to talk about their experiences and will do so, but a child centred focus for interventions limits this: 'Staff needs may be pressing and require attention, but sessions set up by specialists to help staff to help children should not be hijacked to deal with staff members' own difficulties' (Yule and Gold 1993). Staff will not be able to support students if their needs are not addressed. Ignoring teachers' grief has the potential to deprive students of ongoing support and can impact negatively on the school environment and the worklife of teachers.

Conclusion

In conclusion, adopting a comprehensive approach means we accept grief as a life event and as a legitimate area of concern for schools. Rather than seeing loss and grief as a special 'one off' experience it is mainstreamed into educational policy and practice and employment standards, as well as established as a wider health issue, particularly in its links to mental health. The latter area has been identified as a major public health issue in the next 20 years—and within that, depression that is often linked to grief experiences.

From an educational perspective, a comprehensive strategy establishes proactive approaches which assist in:

- creating physical and psychosocial safety;
- demonstrating a school community's caring and responsible behaviour and thereby minimizing litigation threats; and
- helping ensure the public perception of schools as safe, physical, and psychosocial environments.

It is only coordination and cooperation that can create a healing community needed for young people.

There is enough research evidence and collective wisdom to warrant comprehensive action by school communities. However there still needs to be care taken 'to do no harm' and to utilize the technical expertise of bereavement agencies combined with the insight, understanding, and judgement of school personnel. Importantly the voices of young people need to be sought, included, and valued.

References

Averill JR, Nunley EP (1988). Grief as an emotion and as a disease: a social-constructionist perspective *Journal of Social Issues* **44**:79–95.

Corr C, Balk D (ed.) (1996). *Handbook of adolescent death and bereavement*. New York: Springer.

Doka K (1989). *Disenfranchised grief. Recognising hidden sorrow*. Lexington, MA: Lexington Books.

Doka K (2002). *Disenfranchised grief. New directions, challenges and strategies for practice*. Champaign Ill Research Press.

Glassock G, Rowling L (1992). *Learning to grieve. Life skills for coping with losses*. Newtown Millennium Press.

Kauffman J (1989). Intrapsychic dimensions of disenfranchised grief. In: K Doka (ed.), *Disenfranchised grief. Recognising hidden sorrow*, pp. 25–30. Lexington, MA: Lexington Books.

Martin TI, Doka KJ (2000). *Men don't cry...women do: transcending gender stereotypes of grief*. Philadelphia, PA: Bruner Mazel.

Petersen S, Straub RL (1992). *School crisis survival guide. Management techniques and materials for counsellors and administrators*. West Nyack, NY: Centre for Applied Research in Education.

Pfefferbaum B, Nixon SJ, Tucker PM *et al.* (1999). Posttraumatic stress responses in bereaved children after the Oklahoma City bombing. *Journal of the American Academy of Child and Adolescent Psychiatry* **38**:1372–9.

Rowling L (1995). Disenfranchised grief of teachers. *Omega. Journal of Death and Dying* **31**:317–29.

Rowling L (1996). A comprehensive approach to handling sensitive issues in schools with special reference to loss and grief. *Pastoral Care in Education* **4**:17–21.

Rowling L (1999). The role of policy in creating a supportive social context for the management of loss experiences and critical incidents in school communities. *Crisis, Illness and Loss* **7**:252–65.

Rowling L, Holland J (2000). Grief and School Communities: The impact of social context, a comparison between Australia and England. *Death Studies* **24:**35–50.

Rowling L (2002). Youth and disenfranchised grief. In: K Doka, *Disenfranchised grief. New directions, challenges and strategies for practice.* Champaign Ill Research Press.

Rowling L (2003). *Grief in school communities: effective support strategies.* Buckingham: Open University Press

Sheehan M, Cahill H, Rowling L *et al.* (2002). Establishing a role for schools in mental health promotion: The MindMatters project. In: L Rowling, G Martin, L Walker (ed.), *Mental health promotion and young people: concepts and practice.* Sydney: McGraw-Hill.

Silverman PR, Worden JW (1992). Children's reactions to the death of a parent in the early months after the death. *American Journal of Orthopsychiatry* **62:**93–104.

Smith S, Pennells M (1995). *Interventions with bereaved children.* London: Jessica Kingsley.

Stevens M, Dunsmore J (1996). Adolescents who are living with a life-threatening illness. In: C Corr, D Balk (ed.), *Handbook of adolescent death and bereavement.* New York: Springer.

Yule W, Gold A (1993). *Wise before the event. Coping with crises in schools:* London: Calouste Gulbenkian Foundation.

Zisook S (ed.) (1987). *Biopsychosocial aspects of bereavement.* Arlington, VA: American Psychiatric Press.

Chapter 12

Brief interventions in critical care environments

Peter Speck

Introduction

Family structures and attitudes regarding children and death have changed enormously over the past 100 years. Victorian art frequently depicts children involved in death-bed scenes and the funeral processions. The funerals were often of children under 15 years of age and, therefore, it is the siblings that may be seen carrying the baby coffin or walking with the parents to the graveside. In recent times, however, there is a tendency to be protective of young children and the attempt to shield them from the reality of death. This can lead to their being excluded from the 'death' event, seeing the body subsequently and sometimes, the funeral itself. The consequences of such 'protectiveness' can be far reaching for some people and lay the foundations for a variety of problems in later life; especially, if the death is sudden and unexpected.

In 1941, two sisters, aged 6 and 7 were collected from school by their aunt. She told them their mother was ill and they were to spend a few days with her (their aunt and uncle). The girls' father had died some years ago and the uncle was their mother's brother. Nothing was said about the mother's illness. The household was somewhat Victorian and children were seen and not heard, and certainly did not ask probing questions. Two days later, the 7-year-old was helping to make beds when the aunt said, 'I have to tell you—your mother has died'. No further information was given. The little girl was stunned and went downstairs to find her sister. Walking through the kitchen she saw her uncle at the table 'looking like a statue but with tears on his face'. Neither girl felt they could ask for details and at lunchtime the aunt said, 'Your uncle and I have talked this through and you will both have to come and live with us. This will be your home from now on'. The girls were well cared for, and at the age of 11, went to boarding school. Over 60 years later, the elder girl described to me how it was at boarding school that they found a safe space to explore and find out something of what had happened. Their mother had died in hospital, from smoke inhalation and burns, following a fire in the girls' home. While the aunt and uncle were caring, the girls had learnt that one contains emotion and distress and re-engages as quickly as possible with life. They had not attended the funeral and even now, 60 years later, the older sister finds it difficult to cope with deep emotion and threatening experiences.

Ten years later, little work had been done to try and understand the effect of loss on young children. Health professionals frequently perceived the hospitalized, withdrawn child-patient as compliant and 'content', and while the work of Robertson (1952) was initially received with scepticism, it did indicate that the young child's quietness was often an indication of traumatization. Staff training seemed to contain little understanding of the impact of death on the young child.

At the age of 9, in the 1950s, I was a long-stay patient in a TB sanatorium. In a side room I was strapped on my back with suspected TB spine. Another boy R was in the opposite room and, when the doors were open, we could talk, swap comics and games, and develop a friendship over several months. 'R's' condition deteriorated and he developed tubercular meningitis. I watched his decline and vividly remember the hot sunny week when his mouth and lips were bathed in gentian violet to detract the flies that seemed drawn to him. One afternoon, I noticed his breathing change and he seemed to be struggling for breath. I shouted for a nurse and while I waited, R stopped breathing and I was sure (rightly) that he had died. When the nurse arrived, I said that I thought R had died. She dashed into his room then came back and said, 'You're a very wicked boy to have been watching' and shut the door of my room leaving me alone with my distress at the death of my friend, and with the fear that this disease, which we shared, might also kill me. Fortunately, my own parents had a different approach to death and when my uncle had died, a few years ago, I had had the opportunity (aged six) to go and see and touch 'Uncle Fred' and realize a dead body was not frightening and that the Uncle Fred I had known was no longer in that body. The adults in the hospital did not have this understanding and nobody attempted to find out what I had seen, felt or feared. The long-term effects of this experience became one of the motivating forces for my own entry into the health care arena.

In both of these episodes, a young child learnt that for many adults, death was not to be talked about or acknowledged, and that the associated feelings were not to be expressed. It was unnatural for young children to react to the death of another.

Over the years, attitudes within society have changed. Research has increased our knowledge of the way in which children develop their understanding of the concept of death (see Chapter 2). Pioneer figures include Bowlby (1969), Wolfenstein (1966), Furman (1974), and Caplan (1969). In recent years, the work of Parkes (1996), Parkes et al. (1996), Worden (2003), Stroebe (1993), Walter (1999), and Black (1978) has extended our understanding of how people seek to adjust to major losses in their life and drawn attention to the needs of young children and siblings. Current understanding indicates that children need immediate and honest answers that allow them to share in the family grief. They need to know the truth, communicated with warmth. There should be a willingness to listen and respond to their questions, anxieties, and fears concerning the death. If the child's questions and feelings are postponed or ignored by the adults around, then the child may conclude that she/he may be responsible in some way, or that their feelings are unacceptable and push them underground.

Current research findings have not always filtered through to the general population. In my role as a health care chaplain, I have frequently needed to enquire of parents and families whether they have thought about what to say to the children following a traumatic death of a baby, an older sibling, or an adult. Not infrequently, the response has been 'they are too young to understand' or 'It would be too upsetting for them at their age', and we have then begun an exploration together of what the surviving child may or may not already know, and what their needs might be in this situation. In this chapter we shall look at a small selection of situations where the needs of children have been addressed, following sudden unexpected death in an acute hospital setting and highlight some of the key elements in trying to minimize the risk of a complicated grief outcome.

Pregnancy loss

Most Acute Trust hospitals in the UK have developed policies, quality standards, and designated members of staff who can offer advice and support to couples who are facing pregnancy loss. This may be because of spontaneous abortion (miscarriage), termination of the foetus following diagnosis of genetic or other abnormality, or for non-therapeutic reasons. It may be towards the end of the pregnancy when complications occur and the mother has an intra-uterine death or when the live baby is stillborn. In each of these situations, there will be a varying degree of opportunity to prepare those most involved with the pregnancy. The work of such groups as SATFA (Support After Termination for Foetal Abnormality) and SANDS (Stillbirth and Neonatal Death Society) have had a key role to play in helping professional health care staff to assess sensitively the needs of the family, enable them to address the reality of the event, create appropriate memorialization, and obtain on-going support as appropriate. The siblings of the unborn child often have knowledge of the impending arrival of a new brother or sister and may well have experienced natural sibling rivalry. This may not be mentionable to parents, especially if the parents are distressed about the actual or impending loss. If the death of the baby is not referred to, young children can be left wondering if their rivalrous thoughts have been powerful enough to kill the baby.

Distinguishing reality from fantasy can be difficult even for older children, let alone the very young. It is therefore important that there is some exploration with the mother (and father) about what the other children may already know and feel about the new baby and the mother's admission to hospital. This exploration needs to extend to include those siblings without demanding too much of them.

If the loss has not yet occurred, there can be discussion of attitudes and feelings regarding seeing the dead foetus/baby. There is a difference between 'providing opportunity' and implying an 'ought to do'. This relates to viewing, photographs, attending funerals, creating memory boxes, etc. It is especially important to be sensitive to cultural issues, which may not always match a more general expectation based on the family's religious affiliation. A family from Nigeria, who happen to be Christian, may want nothing to do with the dead child because, as one father told me, 'We have nothing to do with dead babies. They are simply passing through here and we let them go'. To encourage a mother to see, touch, and photograph her dead baby might, therefore, be encouraging her to go against the cultural norms of her family.

Many parents recognize the significance of giving their other children opportunity to be involved as far as they wish. It is important that the children are prepared for what they will see as many would have never seen a dead person of any age. Bringing the baby suitably dressed and wrapped into the mother's room in a 'Moses' basket or cot is more natural. The mother may then take the child into her arms and the sibling looks at the child or perhaps takes over the holding of the baby. Talking about the death and the reasons (where known) in a clear and simple way is also important. A member of staff, such as counsellor, midwife, or health care chaplain should be present to 'hold the boundaries' and free the parents to be distressed. The other adult can then be there for the sibling.

Avoid euphemisms and use clear terms such as 'dead', 'died', 'was unable to continue growing inside mummy's tummy' and so on. Frequently, this viewing and examination of the dead baby leads to discussion of what happens to the body now. This may include a post-mortem examination. 'The doctors will wish to examine the baby carefully to see if they can discover why X or Y stopped growing, etc.' 'Then you and your family will need to decide how you want to say "goodbye" to X or Y'. Depending on the age of the siblings, this may lead to discussion of burial, cremation, coffins, putting toys into the coffin, and whether the younger children want, or should, attend. Sensitivity is required to avoid steering people into undertaking activities because 'we' believe they will be good for them. However, people must make an informed choice based on realistic options.

Cot death

Many of the above points apply equally to the distressing arrival of a dead baby in the Accident and Emergency department. The child may sometimes be accompanied by a child-minder, who discovered the baby 'blue' in its pram or cot, or by a distraught parent who has discovered the child dead late at night. In either case, there is the additional complication of a necessary police investigation and coroner's autopsy to ensure that the death is a Sudden Infant Death and not the result of another person's action. The mutual blame that surrounds cot death for many couples is compounded by the necessary coroner's involvement. Sensitivity by the emergency services in undertaking their necessary roles frequently helps to alleviate some of the distress for the parents. Siblings may not always be involved at this early acute stage and may temporarily be cared for by other adults. However, at some point, their feelings and reactions need to be listened to, so that they can be given permission to grieve with the rest of the family and not be shut out. It may be that this is picked up by their having the opportunity to see the dead child in the hospital mortuary viewing room, the A&E department, or at the funeral directors.

Viewing

Two young children, aged five and nine expressed the wish to see their dead baby brother (Mark) who had been stillborn at 26 weeks gestation. The parents thought the 9-year-old boy would cope but were not so sure about his sister. In talking with the 5-year-old, the girl was adamant. 'I know mummy was having a new baby. She's crying because Mark is dead and I want to say goodnight'. It was agreed that chaplain, nurse, parents, and children would go to see the baby. The baby was dressed in a 'Babygro' and placed in a crib. We sat in the waiting area which was a comfortably furnished 'sitting room' environment and discussed what we would see. When the baby was brought to the family, the 9-year-old boy hung back, but the 5-year-old immediately came forward to have a good look. The parents were tearful and seemed unable to respond to the children. The chaplain pointed out features of the dead baby—the dark hair, the finger nails, the nose similar to the little girl. She then said, 'Can I touch Mark?' 'Yes,' the chaplain said. 'Touch his face gently and hold his hand.' She did so and then touched the top of his head. 'It's all squishy,' she exclaimed. 'That's because Mark's head has not grown properly. Now that he's dead, the bones won't join up firmly'. She then touched her head and said 'My head's not squishy'. 'No,' I replied 'that's because you're alive and your head's all joined up'. She then turned to her brother, took his hand, and led him across to the baby and said, 'You feel'. He did so, somewhat apprehensively and then grinned and touched his own head. Finally the little girl said, 'Goodnight Mark' kissed him, and then sat down, sucked her thumb, and hugged her mother. Gradually the rest of the family said their farewells and prepared to leave.

In many ways the 5-year-old led the way and 'managed' the event, but it was crucial that there were people there who could be with the parents and free them to grieve in the presence of the children; while other adults could be there specifically for the children. Again, honesty about the meaning of being 'alive' and being 'dead' in response to the discoveries by the child was important. The key element was being reasonably comfortable with 'death' and 'dead bodies', as a health care professional, together with a willingness to be flexible in response to the young child's wish to lead. Health care staff may feel diffident about encouraging or responding to questions from children about 'death' and 'dying'. Thompson and Payne (2000) indicate that children within the age range of 6–14 years can have a variety of questions to which they would like answers. In particular, they welcome a doctor answering 'how and why' people die. By valuing the child's questions, a doctor can enhance the child's self esteem at a time when children can be feeling especially vulnerable and unable to explore these ideas with other adults who may be too distressed.

Sudden death following a Road Traffic Collision

A family was returning from a holiday along a dual carriageway. It was late at night and pouring with rain. In the car were a husband and wife and their three children—a girl (aged seven) and twin boys (aged five). At a traffic light, the father failed to stop in time and drove into a small lorry crossing the junction. In the resultant crash, the mother was seriously injured and was dead on arrival at the hospital. The father had serious injuries and was admitted to intensive care. One of the twin boys was dead at the scene, the other was injured and in the Accident and Emergency department, his sister with a severe head injury was in the paediatric intensive care. The chaplain on call had been called to A&E to offer support and assistance.

Given that the father and the surviving daughter were unconscious in intensive care, the main focus was the needs and responses of the surviving twin and any other family members. The parents of the wife who had died in the crash had been contacted by the police and were making the 120-mile journey to the hospital. Family Liaison Officers (FLOs) had been assigned to the various people involved in the incident. Their assistance and support over the days and weeks that followed proved to be invaluable (see Chapter 15). The surviving 5-year-old twin was in pain from several fractures, but was becoming more responsive and beginning to ask for his mother. The child (Tom) knew there had been a crash and a big bang, but asked no questions and volunteered no information. It was explained that mummy had been involved in the crash with him and was being looked after in another part of the hospital. The subject of the other family members was not raised at this time. The child's grandmother had relayed a message via the police that she would like to be there when Tom was told more details and it was agreed to wait, if possible, for her arrival.

On meeting, it was clear there was a good relationship between the children and the grandparents. The chaplain, FLO, and A&E staff brought them up to date on the condition of the family survivors. In spite of her own shock and grief, the grandmother still wished to tell Tom about his mother, and she and the chaplain rehearsed how that might be done. They also considered the pros and cons of giving or withholding the news of the other family members. It was decided that they would try to follow Tom's lead rather than push the agenda and risk overloading him. The grandmother also wished her husband and the chaplain to be there with her. The unit had a special paediatric section and this was chosen as an appropriate setting as there were books, games, and pictures to make the whole environment more child-friendly.

Children, like adults, may respond in a variety of ways to news of sudden death: shock and disbelief, 'I don't believe you'. 'You're telling lies', or dismay and protest 'Be quiet! Go away, I hate you!' or withdrawal and apathy, where there may be little response and the adult may desire to re-tell because they don't think they've been heard. In this situation, the child will often look hurt and puzzled by what is happening, but show no emotional response. The child may also quickly switch from the information to wanting to engage with normal activity 'Put the television on' or 'Can I go out to play now', usually dropping their normal 'please' and 'thank you'. It is best if the news is given by a close relative or family member, but, as in this case, supported by someone else who is not quite so emotionally involved or overwhelmed. Health care staff can themselves, of course, feel overwhelmed by identification with the situation and need support before, and debriefing opportunities after, such encounters. Again, clear language of 'dead', 'died', etc. is important and the information should be short and to the point. Amplification of the circumstances can come later in response to questions, or after a period of time to let the first statements sink in.

In the above case, after hugs and kisses from Grandmother, she said. 'Tom, you know you were in a car crash today. I have some very sad and bad news for you. Mummy was badly hurt in the crash and she has died. That's why she isn't here with you now.' There was a stunned silence. Then Tom said 'I WANT mummy NOW.' To which granny replied, 'I know darling, but mummy died in the crash.' Tom then started to cry and the two of them cried together for a while. Tom then said, 'Can I see mummy again?' and granny looked at the chaplain who said, 'When your body is a bit better and you can move around, we could take you to see mummy's body, if you still want to'. Tom then said to granny, 'Will you read me a story?'

It was after the story that Tom said, 'Where is daddy?' and it was explained that daddy and Ruth were in a special part of the hospital having extra special treatment and as soon as possible we would take him to see them. It was then that he mentioned his twin. Grandmother was clearly quite drained by this time and grandfather took over. He followed his wife's earlier lead and reminded Tom of the crash and mother's injuries and death and then said that Tom's brother had also died in the crash. Tom said, 'Does that mean he's with mummy?' Granddad said 'Yes' and Tom replied, 'So, he'll be alright then'.

At this point, the chaplain left them together for a little while, saying that he would be just outside, and reported back to the other key staff what had been happening—and sought personal support from the other team members! Then, a member of the ambulance crew came into the unit with a small teddy bear. She had picked it up at the scene and thought it might belong to one of the surviving children. It turned out to be the dead twin's favourite bear and over the ensuing weeks and months became an important transitional object for Tom and a link to his dead twin brother. The work commenced in the A&E department that evening was only a beginning and over the weeks that followed, the family was kept together as far as possible. Their clinical needs made it difficult initially for them to be in the same unit but as soon as possible they were re-united and cared for in adjacent rooms.

Most Acute Trust hospitals have a Major Incident Response plan which links with that of the emergency services in the community. A part of that plan will usually include a psycho-social response team who will know, and trust, each other through training together and working together. This team will draw upon social work, psychology, psychiatry (adult and child), psychotherapy, bereavement counselling, and chaplaincy input. A major incident is officially 'declared' before the whole team swings into action. However, a crash, such as that described above, is a major incident for the family concerned and, as the de-briefing showed, can impact on a large number of people. In this instance, the chaplain contacted the co-ordinator of the psycho-social response group and together they identified the resources they would need to assess and respond to the needs of this family, while they were in the hospital. It was recognized that the interventions that were possible at this point in their grief were important to minimize the risk of adverse grief later, but would need to lead to longer term care. Therefore the team was also able to review what resources might be available for on-going support after discharge in terms of general support, or more specific referral to a trauma unit, if required. One of the key roles for the chaplaincy in the ensuing weeks was helping the father (an atheist) to consider and plan the funerals. The final choice was a secular funeral, with burial in a woodland burial site, near where the family took their holidays. The funerals were delayed for 10 weeks until all members of the family were well enough to attend. De-briefing was arranged for the A&E staff, the staff on the wards caring for family members, and the members of the emergency services involved at the crash scene (35 people attended). The ripple effect of such incidents, personally and professionally, was graphically demonstrated.

Death of an older child

Sudden death in the teenage years can happen for a variety of reasons. Commonly, it follows trauma, occasioned by road traffic incident, assault, murder, or suicide. It may also be the result of life-threatening disease, where the individual has received treatment and seems to be recovering and then, suddenly collapses and dies. Occasionally the individual has an undiagnosed condition which spontaneously erupts leading to unexpected death, as in the case of sub-arachnoid haemorrhage due to a unknown weak blood vessel in the brain suddenly rupturing.

In all these cases, the admission of the teenager to hospital, and usually intensive care, will also bring a variety of family and friends who will have a wide range of reactions to what has happened. Entering the waiting room of an intensive care unit to explain the likelihood of death, and to support this mixed group of people in their anticipatory grief, can be challenging. One of the most striking things is the recognition that there are various cultural norms operating and the needs of the parents and family members may be very different from those of the sub-culture to which the dying teenager belonged. In order to be sensitive to this, it is frequently necessary to separate out some of the groups, assess the needs, and establish a rapport with each group. A good level of co-operation and communication is required from the health care professionals involved, if the dynamics within and between the groups are to be contained and worked with, in a positive way. A good degree of flexibility in response may also be called for, especially if there is a tendency to apportion blame regarding the lifestyle and influences upon the child who is dying.

Jan was a 17-year-old girl attending six-form college in order to obtain 'A' level exams. Her work record had deteriorated and there were many arguments at home. She stayed out late at night and, at weekends, often stayed overnight at friends. Her younger sister (aged 13 years) was not a confidante and so could shed little light on her lifestyle. Jan was binge drinking and experimenting with a variety of drugs at the weekend. One weekend, her best friend had a bad experience and became very frightened. She asked Jan to go with her to Narcotics Anonymous (NA) and at the meeting, Jan recognized herself. She attempted to follow the programme but not in any serious way. Her parents had no knowledge of this and she was careful to hide her abuse from the family. One evening, she took a lethal mix of drugs and collapsed in a night club. The ambulance took her to the local hospital where, following admission to intensive care, she was put on a life-support machine. Her parents were contacted and arrived at the hospital, with Jan's sister, in a very distraught state. A number of Jan's friends also arrived—to a mixed reception from the parents. Some were school friends who had some idea of Jan's recent habits; others were from the NA group. The clinical picture was poor and Jan had quickly gone into multi-organ failure. A first cycle of brain stem tests was performed and showed that Jan was virtually dead already. A further set would be undertaken the next day before decisions were made with the parents about ceasing life support. The social worker and chaplain assigned to intensive care agreed to work together, with the staff, with the parents, and Jan's peer group. This chapter focuses on the peer group rather than the parents, but clearly the parents' and sister's needs were paramount.

Thinking of the peer group in particular, it was important to try and establish the nature of the relationships and, with the parents' agreement, who should have access to Jan in what were to be her 'last hours'. The parents, in spite of their emotional pain and ambivalence to some of the friends, were generous in allowing access to a group of about eight. Many of the young-sters were genuinely fond of Jan and deeply shocked at the turn of events. Most of them had no religious affiliation but felt the need of help in knowing what to do in the face of impend-ing death. It was important first of all to establish that they were clear regarding the meaning of brain stem death and life support. It was explained that Jan's family were having to face saying goodbye to their daughter and had asked for help in doing that. Her friends might also feel the need for help in saying their goodbyes. Suggestions were made about touching or holding Jan, using her name, saying privately to her some of things they would like to say (or have said earlier), or saying out loud what they felt. They might like to have a brief period of time alone, or together, but they needed to be clear that this was a 'goodbye'. One in the group said that Jan had always wanted to swim with dolphins, but had not been able to. Someone else phoned a brother and asked him to bring a CD of whale and dolphin sounds. With the parents' permission, this was played by the bedside while the various youngsters came and sat or spoke to Jan. Towards the end of the evening, they understood that the remaining time was really for Jan's parents' and family, and it felt important to draw this little group together in some way. Acknowledging that a religious ritual was not appropriate for them, the chaplain suggested that they might like to listen or join in one prayer that he had brought with him. It was the 'serenity prayer' which is used at all NA and AA meetings:

God grant me the serenity

to accept the things I cannot change

to change the things I can

and the wisdom to know the difference.

All of them joined in and some spontaneously held hands. They then hugged Jan's parents and left the unit. The following morning, the repeat neurological tests confirmed brain stem death and Jan's parents asked for life support to cease. The social worker and chaplain were present with the parents at the time Jan died and the parents commented on how moving and sup-portive they had found the group of friends, in spite of their initial feelings of ambivalence and anger at their *assumed* role in Jan's life.

One of the key issues in this situation was working with the different people involved at different levels and, sometimes, as separate groups. Flexibility was also important on behalf of the health care professionals, the staff of the unit, and the chaplaincy which might have been assumed to only be capable of responding in a religious way. Making sure that the clinical picture is clear is vital when there are issues regarding the with-drawal of life support, as many people find it hard to process what they know intel-lectually (that this person has already died—the brain stem has irreversibly ceased to function) from what they feel emotionally (they cannot be dead because they feel warm, the chest is moving up and down, and the heart is beating). Families need time for this processing; especially if the person dying is deemed a suitable candidate for organ donation. The tension between 'head' and 'heart' can be great and different family members and siblings can be at very different points in assimilating what is happening. Clear communication in a compassionate but straight-forward way is crucial. There needs to be relatively good and easy access to the dying person, with overnight accommodation available nearby. Most modern units have addressed these issues in both the design of the unit and the training of staff. Managing oneself in role can be easy or difficult for the health care professional, depending on the circumstances surrounding the death. Sometimes, there are a variety of unconscious 'hooks' which can draw the staff member into an inappropriate level of involvement leading to feeling overwhelmed or actively 'sucked out' of role and ineffective (Obholtzer and Roberts 1987). Recognizing one's limitations and being able to hand over to a colleague from the same, or a different, discipline can be an important strength. Staff support should be a regular part of the life of units which deal with trauma, since you can never predict the cases which will draw you in more than others. Identification with the situation or persons involved in the event can be very powerful and unexpected. The fact that many of Jan's peer group were almost adult, can also hide the fact that this may be the first close encounter with death for many and can trigger off a degree of regression in their behaviour and ability to cope. If offered in the right way, much good learning can occur at such times, which may strengthen their own coping repertoire for the future.

Summary

1. Children do grieve; if adults can recognize this and give them permission.

2. Adults frequently deny the child's grief as a way of protecting the child and themselves from further pain.

3. Children commonly mask their grief and also seek to protect the adult.

4. The experience and expression of their grief is specifically linked to the child's emotional development and cultural patterns within the family and peer group.

5. It is helpful to explore the child's fantasies and magical thinking since these can be sources of guilt and feelings of responsibility for the death.

6. A child's grief may be expressed indirectly through altered behaviour.

7. It is important to respond immediately to the child's grief, accepting their feelings and questions, whatever they may be, with open, honest answers. Care is also needed not to overload the child with information but to proceed at the child's pace. Wanting to pursue 'normal' activities is not necessarily denial but a child's way of trying to digest manageable lumps!

8. Children should be involved, as far as possible, in the grief of the family, the reality of the death, and the funeral.

9. If the child is excluded and feelings become buried or reaction delayed, a complicated grief may ensue requiring additional help at a later point.

Health care professionals involved in the care of children experiencing the sudden death of an adult or sibling need to offer care that is individualized to that child and family and sensitive to the culture and beliefs of that family. Care should also reflect a need for the child's own grief to be valued and expressed without coercion or collusion.

Many bereavement organizations have developed a variety of training opportunities for professionals to enhance their knowledge and skills in supporting families following the death of an adult or a child. Staff have not always availed themselves of such training and the support offered to families has varied considerably. Following the organ retention scandal at Bristol, Alderhey and other hospitals, the Retained Organ Commission in the UK has highlighted the need for Trust hospitals to review their provision for bereavement support in terms of personnel, training, and facilities. The Child Bereavement Trust has identified four main aims for professional staff in framing best practice for the care of siblings and young children:

◆ *To support parents in communicating with their children.* Staff should not be afraid to show compassion for the family and give permission for the expression of grief

◆ *To assist parents in involving their children after a brother or sister has died.* This would also apply if the death was of a parent or other significant adult.

◆ *To ensure the hospital environment is adequate and appropriate.* This relates to bereavement rooms, viewing rooms, chapels, where families may wish to have privacy with the deceased adult or child over varying amounts of time.

◆ *To guide parents in how they can help their children over the subsequent months.* If children cannot express their feelings in words, they may well act out what they feel in 'difficult' behaviour, anger, frustration, or attention-seeking. Children may also become frightened if the surviving adult(s) become ill, in case they also die. Physical affection and routine can become more important at this time. It is also helpful to ensure that the child's school is aware of what has happened, since the child may find it easier to talk to someone outside the home situation. Parents and care-givers must beware the assumption that a satisfactory answer to the child's question 'Where is X or Y now?' is that they have gone to Heaven. Lansdown *et al.* (1997) have shown the complexities of the concepts of Heaven and Hell for children aged 5–8 years. They found that over half declared some belief in Heaven, but with indications that Heaven is not necessarily a pleasant place to be. It is important that we address and attend to the child's anxieties about what happens after death, without planting graphic details that could confuse or frighten the child.

Above all, it is helpful for professionals to remember the words of Bremner (2000)

'Young people are resilient and do grow and develop creatively, if their experiences are acknowledged, their feelings respected, and their questions about death and loss answered. However, with this age group (*she writes of adolescents*) more than any other, the professional has to have the most courage and the least anxiety about getting it wrong. No matter how risky or uncomfortable it feels to us, almost any attempt to communicate and involve the young person is better than exclusion and silence.'

References

Black D (1978). The bereaved child. *Child Psychology* **19**:287–92.

Bowlby J (1969). *Attachment and loss, Vol 1: Attachment.* London: Hogarth Press.

Bremner I (2000). Working with adolescents. *Bereavement Care* **19**(1):6–8.

Caplan G (1969). *An approach to community mental health.* London: Tavistock.

Furman E (1974). *A child's parent dies.* New Haven, CT: Yale University Press.

Lansdown R, Frangoulis S, Jordan N (1997). Children's concept of an afterlife. *Bereavement Care* **16**(2):16–18.

Obholtzer A, Roberts V (1987). *The unconscious at work: individual and organizational stress in the human services.* London: Routledge.

Parkes CM (1996). *Bereavement: studies in adult life,* 3rd edn. London: Tavistock.

Parkes CM, Relf M, Couldrick A (1996). *Counselling in terminal care and bereavement.* Leicester: British Psychological Society.

Robertson J (1952). Film: *A Two Year Old Goes to Hospital.* Tavistock Child Dev. Res. Unit.

Stroebe M, Stroebe W, Hansson R (1993). *Handbook of bereavement: theory, research and intervention.* Cambridge: Cambridge University Press.

Thompson F, Payne S (2000). Bereaved children's questions to a doctor. *Mortality* **5**(1):74–96.

Walter T (1999). *On bereavement: the culture of grief.* Buckingham: Open University Press.

Wolfenstein M (1966). How is mourning possible? *Psycholanalytic Study of the Child* **21**:93.

Worden JW (2003). *Grief counselling and grief therapy,* 3rd edn. London: Brunner-Routledge.

Chapter 13

Working with traumatically bereaved children

William Yule

Bereavement is a part of normal human experience. It is often distressing, and some would say 'traumatic'. For a child to lose a parent or a sibling can radically affect their life. But some deaths are truly traumatic—sudden, unexpected deaths; accidental deaths where the child witnesses the accident; murders, where the child witnesses one parent killing the other. In these circumstances, the child may develop particular stress reactions and depression, as well as bereavement and additional techniques may be required to help the child cope.

Elsewhere in this book, it is argued that the social support from family and friends is one of the most important factors in 'buffering' a child against any adverse effects of a bereavement. Being able to discuss the dead person and their feelings for the deceased in a supportive way is a normal, healthy part of coming to terms with a loss. But when that loss also may have affected the very support systems, then normal healing processes can be interrupted. When the supportive parent is no longer there, when the wider community has been devastated by a disaster, when the incident that caused the death is a horrific accident, then also the wider support systems may be unavailable or dysfunctional.

In such circumstances, the normal processes of grief and mourning may be affected by the experience of trauma. It is widely held that grieving may be inhibited by the stress reactions and that these need to be treated first. As always, there are exceptions to any rule, but this advice seems to hold in general.

So, what are these 'traumatic stress reactions' and how can they be treated so as to permit normal grieving to take place?

Traumatic stress reactions in children

Immediately following a very frightening experience, children are likely to be very distressed, tearful, frightened, and in shock. They need protection and safety. They need to be reunited with their families wherever possible.

Starting almost immediately, most children are troubled by *repetitive, intrusive thoughts* about the accident. Such thoughts can occur at any time, but particularly when the children are otherwise quiet, as when they are trying to drop off to sleep. At other times, the thoughts and vivid recollections are triggered off by reminders in their environment. Vivid, dissociative *flashbacks* are uncommon. In a flashback, the child reports that he or she is re-experiencing the event, as if it were happening all over again. It is almost a dissociated experience. *Sleep disturbances* are very common, particularly in the first few weeks. *Fears* of the dark and bad dreams, *nightmares*, and waking through the night are widespread (and often manifest outside the developmental age range in which they normally occur).

Separation difficulties are frequent, even among teenagers. For the first few days, children may not want to let their parents out of their sight, even reverting to sleeping in the parental bed. Many children become much more *irritable and angry* than previously, both with parents and peers.

Although child survivors experience a *pressure to talk* about their experiences, paradoxically, they also find it very *difficult to talk with their parents and peers*. Often they do not want to upset the adults, and so parents may not be aware of the full extent of their children's suffering. Peers may hold back from asking what happened in case they upset the child further; the survivor often feels this as a rejection.

Children report a number of *cognitive changes*. Many experience *difficulties in concentration*, especially in school work. Others report *memory problems*, both in mastering new material and in remembering old skills such as reading music. They become very *alert to danger* in their environment, being adversely affected by reports of other disasters.

Survivors have learned that life is very fragile. This can lead to a loss of faith in the future or a *sense of foreshortened future*. Their priorities change. Some feel they should live each day to the full and not plan far ahead. Others realize they have been over-concerned with materialistic or petty matters and resolve to rethink their values. Their 'assumptive world' has been challenged (Janoff-Bulman 1985).

Not surprisingly, many develop *fears* associated with specific aspects of their experiences. They avoid situations they associate with the disaster. Many experience 'survivor guilt' – about surviving, when others died; about thinking they should have done more to help others; about what they themselves did to survive.

Adolescent survivors report significantly high rates of *depression*, some becoming clinically depressed, having suicidal thoughts, and taking overdoses in the year after a disaster. A significant number become very *anxious* after accidents, although the appearance of *panic attacks* is sometimes considerably delayed. When children have been *bereaved*, they may need bereavement counselling.

In summary, children and adolescents surviving a life-threatening disaster show a wide range of symptoms which tend to cluster around signs of re-experiencing the traumatic event, trying to avoid dealing with the emotions that this gives rise to, and a range of signs of increased physiological arousal. There may be considerable co-morbidity with depression, generalized anxiety or pathological grief reactions.

Post-traumatic stress disorder – PTSD

Sometimes, these reactions may be both severe and prolonged. Indeed, they may interfere with normal adjustment and development to such an extent that the reaction warrants being diagnosed as a Post Traumatic Stress Disorder or PTSD. The diagnosis of PTSD was first conceptualized in response to observations of Vietnam war veterans presenting with what came to be recognized as a particular pattern of symptoms in three clusters—intrusive thoughts about a traumatic event; emotional numbing and avoidance of reminders of that event; and physiological hyperarousal (APA, DSM-III, 1980). In retrospect, similar patterns were noted as reactions in earlier wars and in prospect, the criteria were adapted, partly operationalized, and applied to adult civilians. Next, the diagnosis was applied to children who had experienced an 'event outside the range of usual human experience... that would be markedly distressing to almost anyone' (DSM-III-R, 1987).

Thus, it was argued that there were certain types of stressful experiences that were very severe and/or unusual and that there was a distinctive form of stress reaction to these. PTSD was classified as an anxiety disorder, but many argued that it should be included as a dissociative disorder. It was increasingly described as 'a normal reaction to an abnormal situation', and so, logically, it was queried whether it should be regarded as a psychiatric disorder at all (O'Donohue and Eliot, 1992).

Results from studies of adults have reasonably established that PTSD, while being predominantly an anxiety disorder, differs from other anxiety disorders in important ways. Thus, Foa *et al.* (1989) showed that the trauma suffered, violated more of the patients' safety assumptions than did the events giving rise to other forms of anxiety. There was a much greater generalization of fear responses in the PTSD groups, and, unlike other anxious patients, they reported far more frequent re-experiencing of the traumatic event. Indeed, it is this internal, subjective experience that seems most to mark out PTSD from other disorders (Jones and Barlow 1992). In adults, the argument is increasingly made that PTSD is an 'abnormal reaction to an abnormal event' that involves a complex interaction of biological, psychological, and social causes (Yehuda and McFarlane, 1995).

Concern has been expressed that the diagnosis is being made too liberally, without due attention being paid to the impact on social functioning. Equally, concern has been expressed that there are other forms of stress reactions to chronic stress as experienced in repeated physical or sexual abuse. Terr (1991), for example, draws a distinction between Type I and Type II traumas, roughly the distinction between acute and chronic.

With its roots in studies of adult psychopathology, the concept has been uneasily extended to apply to stress reactions in children and adolescents. The major difficulty from the outset has been that some of the symptoms are developmentally inappropriate for younger people. Indeed, the younger the child, the less appropriate the criteria.

Many writers agree that it is very difficult to elicit evidence of *emotional numbing* in children (Frederick 1985). Some children do show a loss of interest in activities and hobbies that previously gave them pleasure. Pre-school children show much more regressive behaviour as well as more anti-social, aggressive, and destructive behaviour. There are many anecdotal accounts of pre-school children showing repetitive drawing and play involving themes about the trauma they experienced.

Although parents and teachers initially report that young children do not easily talk about the trauma, recent experience has been that many young children easily give very graphic accounts of their experiences and were also able to report how distressing the re-experiencing in thoughts and images was (Sullivan *et al.* 1991; Misch *et al.* 1993). All clinicians and researchers need to have a good understanding of children's development to be able to assist them express their inner distress.

Scheeringa *et al.* (1995) examined the phenomenology reported in published cases of trauma in infants and young children and evolved an alternative set of criteria for diagnosing PTSD in very young children. Re-experiencing is seen as being manifested in post-traumatic play; re-enactment of the trauma; recurrent recollection of the traumatic event; nightmares; flashbacks or distress at exposure to reminders of the event. Only one positive item is needed. Numbing is present if one of the following is manifested: constriction of play; socially more withdrawn; restricted range of affect; loss of previously acquired developmental skill. Increased arousal is noted if one of the following is present: night terrors; difficulty getting off to sleep; night-waking; decreased concentration; hypervigilance; or exaggerated startle response. A new subset of new fears and aggression was suggested and is said to be present if one of the following is recorded: new aggression; new separation anxiety; fear of toileting alone; fear of the dark, or any other unrelated new fear. To date, these altered criteria have not been tested against the traditional ones. Almqvist and Brandell-Forsberg (1997) provide evidence on how a standard set of play material can be used to obtain objective data on traumatic stress reactions from pre-school children. Thus, one can anticipate a refining of criteria and methods of assessment of PTSD in pre-school children in the next few years.

Incidence and prevalence of PTSD in children

Given that PTSD has only been recognized as occurring in young people since the late 1980s, there are not many studies to inform us as to how common it is. Following the sinking of the Jupiter cruise ship in Athens harbour in October 1988, just over half the teenagers on board developed PTSD, mainly in the first few months. Many others were troubled by partial PTSD and had other disorders such as anxiety and depression (Yule *et al.* 2000). In other words, under certain circumstances, the incidence of PTSD can be high. It does also occur following accidents such as road traffic accidents and the average rate of PTSD in six British studies is around 25–30% (Yule 2000). In many such road traffic accidents, children who survive may aso be bereaved.

However, PTSD is relatively uncommon in the population as a whole. In the recent National Survey of 10 000 British children, the estimated prevalence rate was around 1% (Meltzer *et al.* 2000).

Long term outcome

When PTSD was first described in adults, it was initially assumed that it would not be seen in children and young people (Garmezy and Rutter 1985). This was because up until that time, hardly any clinical researchers had asked children directly about the largely inner distress they were experiencing. Instead, they had interviewed parents and teachers, and, as we now know, children do not often confide their worries in adults who, in turn, grossly underestimate the levels of distress.

Thus, studies like those of the survivors of the Jupiter shipping disaster, by using well-standardized diagnostic techniques clearly demonstrated that PTSD can be a significant consequence of a life-threatening experience. Moreover, the 7-year-follow-up of the Jupiter survivors discovered that a significant minority of children still met strict criteria for a diagnosis of PTSD. Some 17% still had it.

For the purposes of the present chapter, the 33-year-follow-up of the people who survived the coal tip disaster of Aberfan is even more relevant (Morgan *et al.* 2003). Coincidentally, also on the 21 October, but in 1966, just as school was starting, the tip slid down the Welsh mountainside engulfing the school and killing 116 children and 28 adults. One hundred and forty three primary school children survived, but scarcely a family in that tightly knit community escaped the aftermath of the disaster. When re-examined, 33 years later, 29% of the survivors still had PTSD.

Aberfan was an horrendous accident which clearly had long term consequences. It was partly as a result of helping the original survivors that Colin Murray-Parkes developed his ideas on pathological grief reactions. It looks as if a truly overwhelming and life threatening experience which actually involved heavy loss of life, really can lead to long term problems in adjustment. For our purposes, we need to be aware that when a young person is involved in an accident or disaster that also involves loss of life of people known to the young person, then pathological grief reactions may occur.

Assessment

Ironically, while Aberfan was very influential in shaping British views on the needs of the traumatically bereaved, it occurred long before the mental health community had formulated its ideas about PTSD. As was noted above, careful diagnosis involving the use of standard procedures has been influential in getting the nature and extent of the traumatic stress reactions in children fully recognized. With proper assessment and diagnosis, comes better opportunities for effective treatment.

In my own practice, when a child is referred for assessment and treatment, I try to get as much documentation as possible before seeing the child. If the child has been in a relatively public accident, then I may get newspaper descriptions of what happened, television footage, architect's plans, or eye-witness accounts. Then, when I see the child I can anticipate some of his or her story.

On the due date, I will usually see the child with their parents and quite deliberately direct most of my initial questions to the child. I usually ask why they have come to see me and acknowledge that often they may not have wanted to come as they may not want to talk about upsetting things. I explain to them that we have a number of ways of helping children who have been in bad accidents get over their reactions, but that to be able to do so, I need to talk with the child alone about what happened and how they have been feeling, and I also need to talk to their parents about how they were before the accident and how they are now. I then say to the child, 'So, who do you want me to talk to first?' I address this to the child to give them some control over the situation, as experience has shown that many children feel totally out of control of all that is happening to them, and this is a first step in returning some semblance of control to them.

When I see the parents, I normally obtain a standard family, personal, and developmental history; an account of what happened in the incident; and an account of how the child currently behaves. I will follow a standard interview schedule such as the PTSD component of the Anxiety and Depression Interview Schedule for Children (ADIS-C; Silverman and Albano 1996).

When I see the child alone, I spend a few minutes talking to them about themselves, their school, their friends, their likes and dislikes. I remind them that they have come to see me because something scary happened to them and so after a very few minutes I ask them if they are ready, and say, 'Now, tell me about it'. The next thing I usually have to say is, 'Please slow down because I cannot write all of this down'. It has been my experience over the years that when you show children respect and indicate that you are there to take them seriously, then they are amazing in being able to recall, not only what happened, but also how they were feeling then and subsequently. At a suitable point, I ask children who are old enough to read independently, to complete a few questionnaires on traumatic stress symptoms, anxiety, depression, and traumatic grief. This helps in the diagnosis as well as provides a baseline against which response to treatment can be measured.

Sometimes, and especially with younger children, it can be helpful to ask them to draw a bit of what happened or to act it out with toys. One protocol that describes such an approach is that by Pynoos and Eth (1986). Note that one is not 'interpreting' what the child draws; but it can be easier for children to talk about what happened when they are drawing, or acting it out with miniature people, or other toys.

Often, parents relate that their child has changed dramatically, but that they do not know what they are thinking or feeling, because they are too scared to talk to them about it, in case it upsets them further. The parents may be aware that their child wakes in the night, but not aware of the content of any bad dreams. They may notice that the child is distracted during the day, but may not be aware that the child is having intrusive thoughts and images of the accident.

Even in this initial assessment, then, the opportunity presents to educate the parents and the child as to the nature of stress and grief reactions. I let parents know that it is common for children to find it difficult to confide in parents, especially as they do not want to upset them. When, as frequently happens, the child gives me a graphic picture of what they had witnessed and what they thought was going to happen to them, as well as how they are currently feeling. I will ask the child if it would be alright to tell their parents all that as well. Most children are happy for me to let their parents know and often, I am able to facilitate the child talking about their experiences directly with their parents before the close of this initial session.

Witnessing father killing mother: a particular form of traumatic grief

Domestic violence remains a major source of distress and psychopathology in children in the 21st century. Much of the violence is related to rows about money, exacerbated by misuse of alcohol. Until recently, the police regarded 'domestics' as private matters between consenting adults. Within these tempestuous marriages, young children often witness the violence and may even be its target. Many young children, being the centres of their own developing worlds, blame themselves for what they see. They being small and powerless cannot intervene to protect their parents.

Harris-Hendriks *et al.* (2000) have estimated that in England and Wales, every year, some 50 children are orphaned when one parent kills the other—most commonly, the father killing the mother. As a result of their clinical expertise, they were able systematically to report on over 400 children and their study is a model of how a good and careful clinical investigation can contribute substantially to our knowledge.

When the death is discovered, the alleged perpetrator is taken into custody. The house is sealed off as a 'scene of crime'. Someone has to look after the child or children who may have been the only witnesses to what happened—but who is going to do so, even on a temporary basis? If the child is looked after by a paternal relative, they may try to blacken the mother's character to justify what the father did; if a maternal relative takes over, the child hears how dreadful their father is. The child gets caught between these two very emotional sets of relatives. Neither parent is there to comfort the child, let alone begin to explain anything. It can even be that the child has none of their favourite toys or comforters, if they remain at the scene.

Moreover, as a potential witness, the police would want to take evidence from the child as soon as practicable. Even though the Crown Prosecution Services advice on 'Achieving Best Evidence' nowadays allows the interviews to be taped and, if necessary, presented as evidence-in-chief (so that the child does not have to appear in the court), it is still a potentially distressing experience.

At the same time, if it is decided that the child should be placed in the care of the local authority, and usually with foster carers, the child has to adapt to new carers who did not know their parents. Often, in my experience, such carers feel inhibited about helping the child talk about what had happened. If the child has nightmares about blood, what should the carer say? If the child talks about the stabbing, should they ignore it or help the child clarify what happened? This is the sort of scenario that is often presented at the Child Traumatic Stress Clinic.

Two examples; both of them based on real cases, but anonymized serve to illustrate the issues and the way we work.

Case One

Harry: I received an urgent request from a social worker who had been allocated Harry, a $3^1/2$ year old boy, who had been found covered in blood, sitting next to his dead mother. The father had been arrested and later charged with her murder. The killing had occurred less than 48 hours previously, and the social worker asked whether I could provide therapy for Harry.

I immediately and clearly said, 'No'. That was not what the little boy needed most at this point in time. Until he was settled in a good permanent placement and the court case settled, there was little point in embarking on any formal 'therapy'. Rather, I was very happy to consult with his foster carer as to how she was managing the little boy and to advise her on any concerns she had.

Case One—Cont'd

So it was that I met with the foster carer and Harry on a few occasions over the next year. Not surprisingly, given the background of violence, Harry had been neglected and had not reached many of his appropriate social milestones. With firm, loving care, he quickly settled in the foster home. He was able to talk about his mum and a little about what he had seen. He was reassured that what his dad had done was not Harry's fault.

The foster carer became attached to Harry and likewise Harry to her, but she was due to retire and so the Child Care proceedings were initiated and Harry was freed for adoption. By then, he was much more settled and was making good progress at nursery school.

At their request, I met with the prospective adoptive parents and discussed with them some of the issues they might have to face in the future with Harry. He would have the need to revisit his understanding of what happened at various points throughout childhood and adolescence. It may be that various things might unexpectedly trigger distressing reactions and recollections, and that he may need help managing them. Thus, they should enquire about the availability of Child and Adolescent Mental Health Services in their area, so that should Harry get upset, some help could come quickly, bypassing any waiting list.

There are times when specialist 'therapy' is best placed in reserve so that normal healing processes can occur. But specialist therapy does have a role to play.

Case Two

Mary: Mary was a 5$^1/_2$ year old girl when her carer contacted me. She had become hysterical at primary school when she fell and grazed her knee and saw blood. The teachers were unable to console her, even though they had been aware of her recent history.

When I saw her two days later, Mary turned out to be a very articulate young lady. She told me in considerable detail how she had been in bed one night when she heard her parents arguing—nothing unusual. She crept downstairs and saw daddy stabbing mummy. She told daddy to stop but it didn't work, and mummy stopped talking. There was blood all over the place. When the police came, she was taken out through a back way so that she wouldn't see her mother's body—but, of course, she had already seen it and the images were seared into her memory. She spent two nights with her extended family before moving to live with her carer.

The situation was complicated by the feuding within the extended family and that made it difficult for Mary to feel safe and secure. Gradually, she told more about what she remembered. At first, she had mentioned something about a warm drink in her room. It was clear that this was significant to her, but neither I nor her carer could understand how, until it emerged that she thought that if she had not asked for a drink, then mummy would not have gone downstairs and dad would not have stabbed her. Mary being bright, assumed that she was somehow responsible for all this. We reassured her that she was not and told her about dad's drinking habits and the long history of threats which had nothing to do with her. We made sure that both during sessions and at home, she had plenty of opportunity to talk about her mother, see her photograph, and visit her grave.

Case Two—Cont'd

She also suffered from bad dreams—sometimes non-specific monsters chasing her, and at other times very vivid fragments of what she had seen. We reassured her that these were just memories and that they could not hurt her. We placed a 'dream catcher' over her window and she liked the idea of good dreams being recycled and bad dreams being drained away. Gradually, her sleep pattern improved.

Thus, we tackled both her traumatic stress reactions and her grieving in parallel. The picture grew even more complicated when her father was found not guilty of murder, but guilty of manslaughter having pled provocation. Like most convicted men, he received a short sentence and assumes that he will be out in less than three years and resume his paternal duties!

As Harris-Hendriks *et al.* (2000) point out, this is not necessarily a healthy prospect for a child, who not only witnessed her father kill her mother, but is quite adamant that she does not want to see her father at all. The Children Act placed emphasis on the responsibilities of parents, but almost at the cost of the rights of the child. Many of us working in this area would like to see the Courts use Wardship more frequently, so that the children's needs are placed first.

It is not easy to sit there watching children play with toy animals, or draw pictures of home and tell in vivid detail the horrors of what they saw. But they did see it all; I did not. I can show them the respect of listening carefully and let them talk without getting upset. I can slip in advice about how reminders will happen whether they want it or not, and how they can control some of the images that would otherwise frighten them. Above all, once they are in a secure home, I can reassure them that such an incidents will never happen again.

Of course, with older children, there are other, more formal approaches to treatment, some of which my colleagues and I have pioneered.

Crisis intervention

In some ways, the case of Harry illustrates one sort of crisis intervention—a rapid response to a request for help and advice to carers on giving support. It would be good to think that early intervention managed to prevent the development of the worst traumatic stress reactions, but sadly, there is insufficient evidence to be clear about this. Indeed, there has been quite a heated debate in the adult literature which suggests that some early interventions may stop normal healing processes taking place. We should be clear that the literature, flawed and incomplete as it is, does not address traumatic grief or even children.

Having acknowledged that, my own view is that when a traumatic death occurs, there are things that can be done almost immediately, although not necessarily direct with the child. The child needs safety and security. They should have as many personal possessions available as possible. In particular, they should have access to photos of the dead parent. Clear decisions need to be taken about whether or not they should visit the perpetrator in prison—and if so, then never be left unsupervised. Arrangements should be made for them to attend the funeral and participate appropriately to their age. Once settled, additional therapy should be considered. If of school age, then liaising with the teachers is vital to explain why the child may have problems concentrating, why they may breakdown when something in a lesson reminds them of what happened. The child may need to be given an acceptable cover story to explain to others what happened.

If one is faced with a group of children witnessing the death of a school friend or a teacher, then it makes sense to see the whole group together. An initial, structured meeting, a few days after the death, can be very helpful in clarifying to children what had actually happened. It is characteristic of sudden traumatic events, that memory may be vivid, but also patchy. By helping children share their memories as well as their reactions, this can place the event in a better context. It can also be reassuring to learn that others do experience similar, strange reactions.

Note as discussed earlier, the evidence for this preventing later problems is scanty. There should not simply be a one-off 'debriefing' meeting, but rather such a structured meeting should be the start of a planned surveillance and a longer term set of interventions (Yule and Gold 1993). A format for conducting such an initial meeting in a school is described in Dyregrov (1991) and further suggestions for group leaders are in Dyregrov (2003).

Individual treatment

As with adults (Foa *et al.* 2000), there are only two forms of individual therapy which have sufficient evidence base to warrant being used to treat PTSD in children. These are Cognitive Behaviour Therapy (CBT) with prolonged exposure and Eye Movement Desensitization and Reprocessing (EMDR).

CBT

Derived from behavioural and cognitive models of PTSD, the core of CBT treatment is the use of imaginal and in vivo exposure techniques within a safe therapeutic environment (Keane *et al.* 1985) to allow adequate emotional processing of traumatic memories (Rachman 1980). The problem for the clinician is how to help the child remember and re-experience the event and the emotions it engenders in such a way that the distress can be mastered rather than magnified. This will depend foremost on the establishment of a safe and trusting environment in which the traumatic event can be remembered and discussed. Therapists must be prepared to ask children about the most difficult aspects of the traumatic experience, but at the same time ensure that exposure to traumatic memories is paced in such a way that the child does not experience overwhelming anxiety. For many children, talking directly about the traumatic event may be too difficult, and other means of accessing traumatic memories must be found. Asking children to draw their experiences often assist in the recall of both the event and the accompanying emotions (Pynoos and Eth 1986); and with younger children, play may be used (Misch *et al.* 1993).

Imaginal and in-vivo exposure remain core components of CBT. Children are asked to recount what happened to them and to rate how upset they felt during this session. Therapists watch the child closely to note when they might be blocking on particular 'hot spots' in the narrative, and then get back to those parts of the memory. Saigh (1987) was the first to show that, as Rachman (1980) had predicted, longer exposure sessions than normal are needed if desensitization and symptom reduction is to occur. Saigh (1992) has subsequently summarized a five-stage intervention process involving education, imagery training, relaxation training, the presentation of anxiety-provoking scenes, and debriefing, and Saigh *et al.* (1996) have discussed the use of flooding treatment for PTSD in children in greater detail.

The most recent developments have elaborated on the cognitive processing of the emotional reactions, informed by findings from experimental cognitive psychology of memory and emotions. Smith *et al.* (2001, unpublished manuscript) have developed a 10-session CBT Treatment Manual for children and adolescents with PTSD This manual is currently undergoing evaluation as part of a randomized controlled trial by the authors and is broadly based on the cognitive-behavioural model of PTSD, set forth by Ehlers and Clark (2000). The treatment has five main goals:

(1) trauma memories need to be elaborated and integrated into autobiographical memory so that re-experiencing symptoms are reduced;

(2) misappraisals of the trauma and/or of PTSD symptoms need to be modified so that the sense of current threat is reduced;

(3) dysfunctional coping strategies that prevent memory elaboration, exacerbate symptoms, or hinder a reassessment of problematic appraisals need to be eliminated;

(4) maladaptive beliefs of the parents with respect to the traumatic event and its sequelae need to be identified and modified; and

(5) parents need to be recruited as co-therapists.

Very often, as part of the traumatic reaction and of avoidance of reminders of the event, children will have restricted their previous activities. Throughout their treatment they will be encouraged to 'reclaim their lives' by participating in enjoyable activities. These may be set as part of their weekly homework. The exposure part of treatment will usually take the form of imaginal reliving. The child is encouraged not only to tell what happened but also to concentrate on how they felt at the time, what they were thinking, what other sensations they experienced. As their accounts are developed, so they will be more elaborated and the memories put in a correct time-context. The session is audio-taped and the child is given a copy to listen to as a part of between-session home-work. In part of each session, progress is reviewed with the parents and they are given the rationale for each stage of therapy.

EMDR

There is considerable interest and scepticism in Eye Movement Desensitization and Reprocessing (EMDR) treatment (Shapiro 1995). In this paradigm, a child is asked to imagine the worst moment in the traumatic event. Having got the scene firmly fixed in mind, the child is then asked to follow the therapist's fingers as they rhythmically pass in front of the child's face. The child is instructed to let the images change in whatever way happens. In as far as there is any underlying rationale for this treatment, it appears to involve a mixture of exposure and distraction—or 'dual attention' as the Manual prefers. There are other elements to the whole treatment (Morris-Smith 2002). To date, there are no published accounts of randomized controlled trials with children and adolescents. Tinker and Wilson (1999) describe many successfully treated cases but no comparison data are provided. Chemtob *et al.* (1998) used three to six sessions of EMDR with adolescents traumatized following a hurricane and report good results, but again with no control data. Puffer *et al.* (1998) describe a wait list control trial with 20 children who developed PTSD, after a single traumatic event. Over 50% of the children improved from the clinical to non-clinical range on the Impact of Event Scale after only one session of EMDR. As with all techniques that have no clear rationale, caution has to be exercised. However, if symptomatic relief can really be attained in a few brief sessions, then the approach needs to be carefully evaluated. Since there does seem to be a different quality to the memories of a trauma that appear at the same time to be locked in, vivid and unchangeable by merely talking about them, then any technique that will allow emotional processing to proceed must be examined. Yule (2000) describes the successful use of EMDR with two children who developed PTSD following road traffic accidents. More convincing is Ribchester's (2001) account of treating 11 consecutive cases who met DSM criteria for PTSD, identified from an Accident and Emergency department. One child fell out of treatment following a family crisis. In the remaining 10 cases, and with an average of fewer than three sessions, all improved and none continued to meet the diagnostic criteria. Their average scores on all measures improved. But the most exciting finding was that their performances on both the interference and the latency measures on the modified Stroop task normalized, indicating that they no longer showed evidence of selective attention biases to traumatic information.

Concluding comments

The past twenty years has seen a dramatic change in the way traumatically bereaved children are being helped. In the same way that our understanding of bereavement in childhood has improved—as seen in other chapters in this text—our understanding of traumatic stress-reactions has developed rapidly. There is considerable agreement about what stress reactions are shown by children aged 8 years and over. There is still a lot to learn about how they manifest in much younger children. With clearer diagnosis, we have learned that serious stress reactions can be quite common in children following particular traumatic incidents. Even though children can be very resilient, we must not assume that all are, as shown by the longitudinal studies mentioned earlier. For some children, the effects of a traumatic incident can last for many years.

Fortunately, along with better ways of assessing stress reactions have come very powerful ways of treating them too. Compared to the less focused treatments in the past, the new ways are grounded in good theory and evidence of outcome, and are generally fairly brief. Six to ten sessions is the usual duration. Wherever bereavement is involved, this gets more complicated. This is particularly seen in the case when the child loses one, or both parents, and has to be provided a new permanent home. While helping the child to settle in, it may be necessary to postpone active intervention, until the child has settled.

This progress has come about because people have studied the presenting problems and their outcomes in detail. To do this, they had to develop appropriate, brief but valid measures to capture the essence of the child's distress. Measures such as the Child Impact of Event Scale (see www.childrenandwar.org) has made it possible to screen children who can read. Other self-completed measures of anxiety and depression were also very helpful. As yet, there are no similar measures of grief in children, although we are currently developing an inventory of traumatic grief for children and adolescents. Tools to investigate traumatic stress and grief in younger children are needed urgently. As they become available to us, we will be able to test out the best ways of helping children affected by traumatic bereavement.

References

Almqvist K, Brandell-Forsberg M (1997). Refugee children in Sweden: post-traumatic stress disorder in Iranian preschool children exposed to organized violence. *Child Abuse and Neglect* **21**:351–66.

American Psychiatric Association (1980). *Diagnostic and statistical manual of mental disorders*, 3rd edn. Washington, DC: American Psychiatric Association.

American Psychiatric Association (1987). *Diagnostic and Statistical Manual of Mental Disorders*, 3rd edn (revised). Washington, DC: American Psychiatric Association.

Chemotob CM, Nakashima J, Hamada R *et al.* (in press). Brief treatment for elementary school children with disaster-related posttraumatic stress disorder: a field study. *Journal of Clinical Psychology*.

Dyregrov A (1991). *Grief in children: a handbook for adults.* London: Jessica Kingsley.

Dyregrov A (2003). *Psychological debriefing: a leader's guide for small group crisis intervention.* Ellicott City, MD: Chevron.

Ehlers A, Clark DM (2000). A cognitive model of posttraumatic stress disorder. *Behaviour Research and Therapy* **38**:319–45.

Foa EB, Steketee G, Olasov-Rothbaum B (1989). Behavioral/cognitive conceptualizations of post-traumatic stress disorder. *Behavior Therapy* **20**:155–76.

Foa EB, Keane TM, Friedman MJ (ed.) (2000). *Effective treatments for PTSD: guidelines from the International Society for Traumatic Stress Studies.* New York: Guilford Press.

Frederick CJ (1985). Children traumatized by catastrophic situations. Ch 4 in S. Eth R. Pynoos (ed.), pp. 73–99. *Post-Traumatic Stress Disorder in Children.* Washington: American Psychiatric Press.

Garmezy N, Rutter M (1985). Acute reactions to stress. In M Rutter, L Hersov (ed.), *Child and adolescent psychiatry: modern approaches* 2nd edn, pp. 152–76. Oxford: Blackwell.

Harris-Hendriks J, Black D, Kaplan T (2000). *When father kills mother,* 2nd edn. London: Routledge.

Janoff-Bullman R (1985). The aftermath of victimisation: rebuilding shattered assumptions. In CR Figley (ed.) *Trauma and its wake,* vol 1, pp. 15–35. New York: Brunner/Mazel.

Jones JC, Barlow DH (1992). A new model of posttraumatic stress disorder. In: PA Saigh (ed.) *Posttraumatic stress disorder: a behavioral approach to assessment and treatment,* pp. 147–65. New York: Macmillan.

Keane TM, Zimmering RT, Caddell JM (1985). A behavioral formulation of PTSD in Vietnam veterans. *Behavior Therapist* **8**:9–12.

Meltzer H, Gatward R, Goodman R *et al.* (2000). Mental health of children and adolescents in Great Britain. London: The Stationery Office.

Misch P, Phillips M, Evans P *et al.* (1993). Trauma in pre-school children: A clinical account. In: G Forrest (ed.) *Trauma and Crisis Management.* ACPP Occasional Paper.

Morgan L, Scourfield J, Williams D *et al.* (2003). The Aberfan disaster: 33-year follow-up of survivors. *British Journal of Psychiatry* **182**:532–6.

Morris-Smith J (ed.) (2002). EMDR: Clinical applications with children. Association for Child Psychology and Psychiatry, Occasional Paper No. 19.

O'Donohue W, Eliot A (1992). The current status of post-traumatic stress disorder as a diagnostic category: problems and proposals. *Journal of Traumatic Stress* 5:421–39.

Puffer MK, Greenwald R, Elrod DE (1998). A single session EMDR study with twenty traumatized children and adolescents. *Traumatology*, 3(2), Available on the internet: http://www.fsu.edu/~trauma/v3i2art6.html

Pynoos RS, Eth S (1986). Witness to violence: The child interview. *Journal of the American Academy of Child and Adolescent Psychiatry* 25:306–19.

Rachman S (1980). Emotional processing. *Behaviour Research and Therapy* 18:51–60.

Ribchester T (2001). Examining the Efficacy of EMDR as a Treatment for PTSD in Children and Adolescents. Unpublished D.Clin Psychol Thesis, University of London.

Saigh PA (1987a). In-vitro flooding of an adolescent's posttraumatic stress disorder. *Journal of Clinical Child Psychology* 16:147–150.

Saigh PA (1992). The behavioral treatment of child and adolescent posttraumatic stress disorder. *Advances in Behaviour Research and Therapy* 14:247–75.

Saigh PA, Yule W, Inamdar SC (1996). Imaginal flooding of traumatized children and adolescents. *Journal of School Psychology* 34:163–83.

Scheeringa MS, Zeanah CH, Drell MJ *et al.* (1995). Two approaches to the diagnosis of postttraumatic stress disorder in infancy and early childhood. *Journal of the American Academy of Child and Adolescent Psychiatry* 34:191–200.

Shapiro F (1995). *Eye movement desensitization and reprocessing: basic principles, protocols and procedures.* New York: Guilford Press.

Silverman WK, Albano AM (1996). *Anxiety disorder interview schedule for DSM-IV: Child and parent interview schedule.* San Antonio, TX: The Psychological Corporation.

Smith P, Dyregrov A, Yule W *et al.* (1999). *A manual for teaching survival techniques to child survivors of wars and major disasters.* Bergen, Norway: Foundation for Children and War.

Smith P, Perrin S, Yule W (1999). Therapy matters: cognitive behaviour therapy for post traumatic stress disorder. *Child Psychology and Psychiatry Review* 4:177–82.

Smith P, Perrin S, Yule W *et al.* (unpublished manuscript). Cognitive-behavioral therapy for childhood posttraumatic stress disorder: treatment manual. Department of Psychology, Institute of Psychiatry, London.

Sullivan MA, Saylor CF, Foster KY (1991). Post-hurricane adjustment of preschoolers and their families. *Advances in Behaviour Research and Therapy* 13:163–71.

Terr LC (1991). Childhood traumas—An outline and overview. *American Journal of Psychiatry* 148:10–20.

Tinker RH, Wilson SA (1999). *Through the eyes of a child: EMDR with children.* New York: Norton.

Yehuda R, McFarlane AC (1995). Conflict between current knowledge about posttraumatic stress disorder and its original conceptual basis. *American Journal of Psychiatry* 152:1705–13.

Yule W (2000). Treatment of PTSD in children following RTAs. In: E Blanchard, E Hickling (ed.), *Road accidents and the mind*, pp. 375–87. Oxford: Elsevier Science.

Yule W, Bolton D, Udwin O, *et al.* (2000). The long-term psychological effects of a disaster experienced in adolescence. I: the incidence and course of post traumatic stress disorder. *Journal of Child Psychology and Psychiatry* 41:503–11.

Yule W, Gold A (1993). *Wise before the event: coping with crises in schools.* London: Calouste Gulbenkian Foundation.

Chapter 14

Helping the family following suicide

Kari Dyregrov and Atle Dyregrov

Introduction

Even if someone had dropped an atom bomb in the middle of our community centre, we could not have been more affected…

(A father speaking 1½ years after losing his 14-year-old son by suicide)

The following chapter describes how the life of parents and children, and the family as a whole, is affected by the suicide of a parent or sibling. There is also discussion of what support bereaved family members themselves want. The next section examines how family, friends, and colleagues may assist. Finally, suggestions about professional assistance to the family bereaved by suicide will be provided, paying special attention to information and care for children. As children's situations following suicide largely depend on their parents' ability to cope with the loss, this important aspect will be emphasized. Researchers have identified significant associations between the psychosocial features of the children and parental psychiatric symptoms following deaths by suicide.

Individual effects of a suicide

The fact that a parent or sibling chooses to end his or her life is threatening and devastating to those left behind. Parkes (1998) emphasized that in the wake of a traumatic loss such as a suicide, there are possibilities that the grief process can go awry. The word 'trauma' itself indicates that an event is a shock. In addition, there are several other circumstances and qualities associated with suicidal deaths that make them traumatic; they occur suddenly and unexpectedly, there is a perceived lack of control, the events are of out of the ordinary, and they create long-lasting problems. When a family member dies suddenly and unexpectedly by suicide, the experience often results in serious and long lasting psychosocial problems for the close family including children. The traumatic event has the capacity to disturb vital functions within the individual parent or child, or within the family system as a whole. Thus it is important that the impact of this particular mode of death be understood and recognized, in order to respond adequately to those who need help, either on an individual or familial level.

Existential crisis

Janoff-Bulman (1992) concludes that traumatic losses often result in an existential crisis that challenges the bereaved individuals' assumptions of their existence in the world, the safety they had previously taken for granted, and what may possibly happen to them.

The brutal upheaval in the lives of individuals may make great demands on their capacity to confront and handle what has happened, cognitively as well as emotionally. Results from the Norwegian nationwide 'Support and Care Study' (Dyregrov 2003; Dyregrov *et al.* 2003), documented that over one and a half years after the sudden death of an offspring by suicide (< 30 years), bereaved parents reported serious existential, psychological, physical, and social problems.

Post Traumatic Stress Disorder

This nationwide study found that half of those bereaved by suicide suffered from levels of post-traumatic psychological distress indicating risk of PTSD. Common post-traumatic reactions are; unwanted thoughts and images (intrusive reactions), strong anxiety (arousal reactions), as well as denial of the event and its consequences (avoidance reactions). Many also experienced psychic distress such as anxiety and insomnia, or severe depression. Sudden, untimely, preventable, and violent suicidal death may also lead to delayed or distorted mourning; or what is proposed as the syndrome of complicated/traumatic grief (Prigerson *et al.* 2000). These symptoms are distinct from bereavement-related depression. The bereaved are preoccupied with thoughts of the deceased, search and yearn for the person, experience disbelief about the death, are stunned by it, and have difficulties in accepting the death. In our study, 78% of the parents who lost their offspring to suicide scored above the cut-off level for risk of complicated grief at 1 1/2 years following the loss (Dyregrov *et al.* 2003).

Physical illness

A number of studies have documented that traumatic bereavement is associated with physical illness due to pathophysiological changes related to psychological distress. Increased muscular activity may explain why muscular-skeletal problems such as headaches and bodily pain are commonly experienced. Increased susceptibility to infectious diseases, cancer, or diseases of the cardiovascular system is seen after a suicide due to a suppression of the immune system. Another feature is an increase in sick-leave from work and hospital admissions associated with increased physical illness, as well as an increased incidence of early death (Li *et al.* 2003). In the Support and Care Study, 62% of all parents scored above the cut-off score for high levels of psychosocial and physical complaints.

Social difficulties

In addition, the bereaved often experience long lasting social difficulties, for example with their social identity and social relations, as well as problems with social interaction in the family.

As reported in other studies, one of the main findings in the Support and Care Study was that bereaved individuals withdrew and isolated themselves from others (Dyregrov 2003), both from people outside the family, and from each other inside the family. In addition, members of their social network withdrew from them. It seems that those bereaved by suicide become more isolated than other bereaved groups because of stigmatization or 'self-stigmatization', feelings of guilt, shame, anger, rejection, or loss of energy to socialize. Thus the tendency to withdraw from social life may create a feedback loop between social and psychological dimensions. Unfortunately, social and emotional withdrawal often acts as a barrier to accepting offers of social support and professional assistance. The existential crisis that compels the bereaved to reorganize or change their cognitive 'schemas', may lead to a change of attitudes and values that results in changes being made to social life. Such processes may lead to the dismissal of relationships and friends and to less social life. Another explanation for a decline in social interaction may be isolation due to increased physical illness and changes in life events (Dyregrov 2003; Dyregrov *et al.* 2003). In fact, social isolation was the strongest predictor for impaired general health, as well as the traumatic after-effects and complicated grief reactions in our study.

Although children and adolescents usually have a different grieving pattern than adults, they may be struggling with many of the same problems. Research has documented that child and adolescent development may be impeded by the lack of emotional accessibility of parents because of their grief and trauma reactions following suicide. Pfeffer and colleagues (1997) reported that, after a suicide in the family, between 25–40% of children and adolescents fulfil criteria for a diagnosis of PTSD. Another serious consequence is that children and adolescents may suddenly lose an important role model in a sibling or a parent in years of developmental importance. Thus, the suicide may trigger an identity crisis in the youngest members of the family. Enduring guilt, anger and distress, and significant disturbances in self-esteem may increase the occurrence of depression and chronic illness. Children and adolescents who lose a close family member to suicide often drop out of school for a period, or experience academic difficulties. The individual reactions of children must be viewed in a familial and parental context.

Effects of suicide on the family

Communication difficulties

The impact of the suicide on the individual may create a feedback loop between difficulties of interaction and communication often seen within families. The level of communication in the family, and thus the prospects for mutual support within the family system, is closely related to parental attitudes towards the loss. In particular, difficulties between spouses, different grieving patterns, or feelings of guilt or reproach for the death, will impact seriously on the family climate. Common difficulties among partners after the loss of a child by suicide are: fathers' concern and worry about the grief of mothers, the anger of mothers because the fathers do not share their grief, initial breakdowns in communication, loss of sexual intimacy, and general irritability between partners. Different grieving patterns often involve women employing various strategies to confront the loss, whereas men often cope through more avoidant behaviour. Thus, women who wish to talk about and share their feelings about the death may criticize their male partners who instead prefer to work hard. Without knowledge of the most 'typical grieving patterns' of women and men, partners may criticise each other for not reacting appropriately to the loss, for dwelling upon the death, or for lack of understanding. However, it is also important to emphasize that the majority of marital relationships survive the strain brought about by a child's death and may even be strengthened in the long run. Several studies confirm that although some couples are torn apart, most couples stick together (Schwab 1998; Oliver 1999). However, open communication and mutual support within the family seem to be imperative to the individual's and family's integrity following a suicide.

Why?

Feelings of shame, guilt, and blame among the bereaved are likely to lead to avoidant communication patterns. Family members will seek the answer to the question of why the suicide happened. Striving to find an answer, children and adults will often question the extent to which they, or the other surviving family members, contributed to the fatal outcome. Children may believe that their parent abandoned them because of something they did or said. Adolescents may feel intense anger, or blame the surviving parent because they did not do enough to help the parent or sibling who committed suicide. People bereaved by suicide often become obsessed with the 'if onlys' that could have brought about a different outcome. Thoughts that are devastating for the bereaved may seem completely irrational to outsiders. Families who are unable to ventilate or discuss these strong feelings and thoughts within the family need professional help to create a healthier climate for communication.

Change of roles

After the initial shock and distress following the suicide, many caretakers are not able to resume their parenting role or day-to-day activities. This can mean that children's ability to mourn the death and express their feelings and reactions related to the loss is often severely restricted by their concerns for parental welfare. In fact, the demands on the parent(s) may be so great that the needs of surviving children can easily be forgotten or overlooked. Children may undertake the parental role for months, or even years. The adolescents in the Support and Care Study said that they did not blame their parents for overlooking them, but they wished that some adults 'from outside', to whom they did not have to give something back, could have 'looked after' them during the initial months following the sibling suicide.

Moreover, mutual support in the family may be impeded by parents' or children's catastrophic anxiety resulting in exaggerated attention or overprotective behaviour. Well-intended acts of parents, who want to protect their children from pain and sorrow, often worsen the family climate. In line with other studies, our study showed that bereaved children also seek to protect their grief-stricken caregivers, long after the suicide (Rakic 1992; Dyregrov 2001). In order not to stir painful memories and emotions in their parent/parents, children often restrain themselves from mentioning the death or the dead even though this conflicts with their desire to talk. If they express their need for parental support, they may feel guilty about making such demands. One young sibling expressed this when she said:

> If I see that my mum or dad is in a good mood, I don't want to bother them if I feel sad. I don't want to complain and say; 'Oh, I think this is terrible'. If I do, you can see that they start to think of my dead sister immediately. The opposite also happens, if I am in a good mood, and they are sad. Therefore, I usually try to avoid them.

Secrecy about the death or lack of open communication may result in interminable mourning and permit a 'ghost' to become an integral member of the family system. Children and adolescents may have knowledge of previous suicide attempts of siblings that the parents do not share, or the surviving parent may mourn an unresolved conflict that made the spouse kill him/herself. If 'forbidden knowledge' prevents a shared environment of communication and understanding about the suicide, this may nurture problems within the family.

Because the need to understand *why* seems to be especially important following suicide, it may be vital for the family functioning to create a shared acknowledgement of the reality of the death in the family.

A process of reconstruction or re-ordering of meaning seems to be central to healing processes during grief. Thus, the opportunity to express thoughts and feelings about a loss to others may contribute considerably to the healing of the biographical disruption caused by the event (Neimeyer 2000). How well the family manage to communicate about the loss and attend to individual family members will largely depend on the family's pre-existing coping and communication patterns. Under favourable conditions, a bereaved family can shift the roles and relationships within the family to compensate for the loss, and the sharing of grief and pain leads to strengthening of family ties. Research shows that the more expressive and sharing family members are, the closer they feel to one another in the wake of a suicide. Although couples that value open communication may show stronger grief reactions in the first phase after the loss than couples that do not, they seem to cope better over time. 'Disengaged' or 'conflicted' families experience greater distance while cohesive or expressive families report more closeness to one another following suicide. The greater the disengagement and level of conflict the younger members of the family perceive, the more distant they feel from their parents. Conversely, the more expressive and sharing family members are, the closer they feel to one another. Thus, if family members are able to act openly and share feelings and thoughts with each other, they may move through the grieving process within an accepting and supporting family atmosphere. In addition, family recovery will be determined by the interplay of factors such as: nature of the death itself, the family's prior history of trauma and loss, prior and current functioning of the family, family coping resources, and availability of help and support.

Difficulties such as a tendency towards isolation, and family interaction and communication problems following a suicide in the family may necessitate professional assistance. However, it is important to know what kind of help and support the bereaved themselves perceive to be necessary after a suicide in the family.

What kind of help and support do families want?

The mother of a young boy who hung himself exemplifies the desperate need for help following a suicide:

> When you experience such a disaster, you are not capable of asking anyone for anything. You are completely lost in the world and feel like you are drowning, and you need to be held up by someone.

The bereaved in the Norwegian Support and Care Study expressed a strong need for both formal (professional/community based) and informal (social network) assistance in dealing with their loss (Dyregrov 2002, 2003), as others also have found (Murphy 2000; Provini *et al.* 2000). In this section, their wishes for professional assistance will be outlined, mainly voiced by families in our study bereaved by suicide. When asked to describe 'ideal professional help', the bereaved highlighted the following aspects:

They wished for:

- immediate outreach help from trained personnel
- information about the event and reactions that may arise
- various kinds of assistance
- help for bereaved children
- the opportunity to meet with others who have experienced the same or a similar situation
- help over time.

These suggestions about 'ideal patterns of support' are parallel to those expressed within the scarce, prevailing research literature, as well as the general advice from clinicians working in the field of crisis psychology. A large proportion of the bereaved claim that they want more or other types of help than that which they receive, and they ask for systems that will secure automatic contact from a professional team. They ask for stability and continuity in support, competent helpers, and help that is flexible and individually adjusted.

Immediate and outreach help

The bereaved want early community outreach help without having to take the first initiative. They claim that they are not able to ask for the help that they really need, even if helpers tell them to 'contact us if you need help'. Several important reasons may explain why the bereaved do not seek help to the degree that they deem necessary. First, exhaustion and loss of energy make many bereaved people incapable of initiating contact with community services. Thus, paradoxically, one of the reasons why they need help becomes a barrier to obtaining it. A second reason why traumatically bereaved people want to be contacted and offered help is probably due to the pervading stigma of suicide. Internalizations of shame and guilt, and possible prejudice shown by others may also account for their reluctance to seek the help they need. The bereaved family may also not know what kind of professional help they need, or what is available. Well aware of their changing needs for help during the bereavement process, the parents and siblings in our study also emphasized that assistance should be repeatedly offered during the first year. A man gave an example:

If the community health service had contacted us and offered some regular help after the suicide, I could have treated this contact as a life buoy, knowing that it was there, and grabbing it as necessary.

Information

Immediately after the suicide, bereaved relatives often feel a desperate need for different kinds of information. They ask for information on medical aspects of the death, the process of mourning, and possible side effects of the death on family members and family systems. In particular, they ask for advice concerning help for children and difficulties between spouses following suicide in the family. Bereaved families want both verbal information and written information.

Various kinds of assistance

The bereaved families in our study clearly confirmed that the focus of help had not been adequately tailored to all their concerns. Besides psycho-educative information, the parents asked for help with existential, practical, economic, and legal matters, as well as therapeutic interventions and advice. In order to reduce distress, nightmares, flashbacks, etc., more specific psychological help and advice was desired by the parents. This included a wish for 'psychological help' for themselves, their children, and for the family as a whole.

The high incidence of parents at risk of developing complicated grief, PTSD and general health problems in our sample probably indicates that the parents would have benefited from more specific help than they received.

Help for bereaved children

The parents in the Support and Care Study asked for different kinds of advice on how to help and deal with the surviving siblings. Two-thirds of the parents wanted more help for their children, and 45% wanted psychological help, emphasizing the necessity of focusing more on this vulnerable group. Parents also wanted family counselling to increase harmony and resolve conflicts in the parent–child relationship, and to get support for coping with the needs of their child. Bereaved adolescents requested support as separate individuals, and help to prevent them taking on parental roles and responsibilities for younger siblings.

Opportunities to meet with others

Many bereaved want to meet with others who have experienced the same or a similar situation. The bereaved families in our study requested help to mobilize social networks or establish contact with grief groups or organizations for the bereaved. They asked that local authorities should take steps to organize links between those bereaved by suicide, either one-to-one, or in support groups. They emphasized the importance of learning from the unique experiences of other bereaved people concerning 'how to survive the pain'. A woman bereaved by suicide explained:

> Those who have lost someone in the same way as us give a special kind of support. You don't need so many words, because they know what to say and not to say.

Help over time

The duration of follow-up is a central issue, and most of the bereaved claim that an ideal follow-up would need to encompass a lengthy time perspective. The questionnaire data in our study showed that 73% wished they had been offered contact with authorities and, if necessary, help from professionals for at least one year. In the interviews, a high proportion also pleaded for support and help over 'at least two years', or 'as long as it is needed', or 'the rest of our lives'. The reality is that the bereaved are often supported during the first few weeks while they are in shock or busy with the funeral, etc., only to be left alone to face the harsh reality after the first month. Most of the network support also stops after a few months.

Suicidally bereaved families commonly struggle with serious problems for a much longer period than realized both by the health service and social networks. In summary, the bereaved had the following advice for health care professionals about how they could help:

Advice from those bereaved by suicide to health and social care professionals

- Be organized—develop or instigate routines for response;
- Be proactive, don't wait for us to come to you;
- Don't swamp us with help initially and then leave us with nothing;
- Be there when the reality of the death sets in;
- Be flexible—listen to what we need;
- Provide us with information (What will happen? Where and from whom will we get help? What are 'normal' grief reactions—individual, family, gender differences?);
- Help our children and help us to help them;
- Do not forget the extended family;
- Help us get in contact with others who have experienced the same bereavement;
- Be available to us for at least a year.

Immediate help for children

If children are present at the scene when a dead person is found, it is important to limit their exposure to the event, though not by force. They should be led away from the scene, have an adult they trust with them, and have what happened explained to them in concrete terms adjusted to their age and maturity. Do not use phrases such as: 'It will be all right' or 'It could have been worse'. Providing them with information about what will happen in the hours and days to come will be appropriate for school children, while younger children need the presence of an adult to balance the anxiety that witnessing powerful adult reactions to the death can invoke in them. If no one from the family can be with them, a neighbour, adult friend, or other adult they trust (e.g. a teacher) should stay with them until a family member can come.

In the immediate situation, the child will need reassurance that adults they know will be there for them, and that they will not die or take their life as the suicide victim did. It is extremely important to create a caring, safe environment for the child where they can get the support they want, where they can have a lap to sit on and close physical comfort to counterbalance the increased arousal created by the sudden death. They should not, however, be given false assurances or any hope of the person returning or being alive.

Telling a child about a suicide

If the child was not present when the suicide happened or when the body was found, it is important not to postpone telling them what has happened. There are several reasons for this: it will lead to a discrepancy between adult and child knowledge that has the potential for creating distrust when the child realizes that he/she was not told the truth; children overhear what adults talk about and can often understand that there is incongruence between what adults say to one another and what they themselves are being told; others in their social surroundings may learn about what happened and so friends and others may confront them with the truth at a time when adults have no control of the situation or information. Although it may be hard to tell them openly and directly about what happened, this is often harder on the adults who face this task than for the children being told.

Depending on the age and maturity of the child, one has to choose what words to use, what context to place the suicide in, and how much detail one relates. The child does not need to have all the details, but does need to know that the death was caused by the deceased themselves, and how it was done. There is no reason to go into detail, unless being asked directly by the child. If they do ask and it is too difficult to answer, one response could be 'I do not know exactly how to explain this to you. I will think about this and then tell you later today or tomorrow'. This allows time to think and if possible to consult with someone else who knows the child or who has more experience of such situations. If there is a suicide letter it will be important to tell the child about this, even if there is something written that they will not understand until they are older. This should be explained to the child.

It is often difficult to describe the motive for the suicide to a child. It may not even be known. If it is not known it is possible to talk to the child about why people commit suicide and say that one does not know why their parent or sibling did this, but often, it is because people become so sad that they can see nothing to live for.

It is important to convey that the adult did not do this because he/she did not love them, but because things felt so bad for them that not even the thought of the children could keep them from taking their own life. There are various strategies for how to choose to explain a suicide and the strategy, to some extent, must be based on the circumstances of the actual death. When there is a history of depression, we use a metaphor where a person's thoughts are likened to leaves in autumn that wither and die (Raundalen 2000). Such an explanation is, of course, dependent on a history of depression or depressive mood and you must consider the nature of the child and their relationship with the person who died.

Whatever explanation is used, it is important to allow the child to ask questions, and to return to the subject within the first few days to check out what the child has understood. Children may harbour a conviction that their own thoughts or behaviour somehow contributed to the death; so, it is important to tell them that nothing they have done, said, or thought or not done, said, or thought led to what happened.

> When Julia was 12 years old, her mother committed suicide after a long history of being manic-depressive. Her mother used to wave from the window as Julia left for school in the morning, but on the morning of the suicide, she did not come to the window. Julia blamed herself for not having understood that there was something wrong that morning and felt that perhaps if she had returned instead of going to school it would not have happened. She also blamed herself for being 'moody', thus contributing to her mother being sad. Because no one noticed or knew how she blamed herself, it was not until she entered therapy that her self-blame could be addressed through cognitive techniques. She was then able to say: 'Mother was sad from before I was born'. If during the immediate follow-up she had received more reassurance that nothing she did or did not do had anything to do with the suicide, her self-blame might have been prevented

Including children in rituals

Participation in rituals makes the loss real, has great symbolic significance, and provides an opportunity for expression of thoughts and feelings that were provoked by the suddenness of the death. Elsewhere we have written in more detail about how and when to include children in rituals (Dyregrov 1996). We wish to emphasize the importance of including children whenever possible. A child that is only six months of age will not have a conscious experience nor have a memory of being present in the viewing of a father that committed suicide. However, 15 years later, that child is $15\frac{1}{2}$ and it may be very important to learn that 'yes, you were present in the room when we said farewell'.

Viewing the body

Where an adult can view a dead body, there is no reason to exclude a child. It is, however, important to prepare the child properly for the experience. This preparation should include being prepared for sensory impressions (what the room will be like, in what ways the dead person looks different from usual, how they will feel cold if he/she touches them, etc.), how adults or the child themselves may react, and what they can bring to put in the coffin (drawing, letter, other memento). They should also have adult support during the ritual. It may be helpful for someone other than the parent to be present. Following the ritual, children must have a chance to express their reactions and to receive answers to their questions e.g. 'what happens to the body now'?

Talking with children

It is often wise to use open questions in conversations with children, or to ask them to tell you what you have explained to them or to tell you what they have understood about what happened. This can reveal misperceptions and misunderstandings that can be corrected. Initially, it will be important to help the child and other family members to get a 'grip' on what has happened. It may be important to gather and record information which may be significant and hard for the child to find later on. A child has less understanding of the chronology of events and may need special help from adults to organize what happened along a 'time line'. A child will revaluate what happened and their own involvement in what happened as they grow older, and have a fuller understanding of the long-term consequences of the event. Children process such a loss over time with seemingly little attention to the death for periods of time punctuated by periods of active processing. Interventions can therefore be brief and focused on the issues concerning the child at the time.

Information for adults

To help children cope with what happened, it is important that the parents, the surviving parent, or other caretaker, receive adequate assistance to help them care for their children.

Adults need to understand:

- how children react to death;
- how important it is that children get honest information about what has happened and what will happen in the near future;
- what children understand at different stages of their development;
- how they cope with grief;
- that children may:
  - need to sleep in their parent's bedroom for a time;
  - become more clingy for a period;
  - behave as if nothing has happened;
  - need stability in daily routines.

It may be difficult for an adult overwhelmed by what has happened to talk with children about what is most painful. From our clinical work we know that children often refrain from talking about their loss because they sense that their parents or remaining parent easily become upset or that it causes them pain. For this reason, it is important that other adults are there for them if they want to talk about their longing or pain related to the loss. If the child has been present at the death, it will be important for them to be able to talk about their sensory impressions—the sights, smells, and sounds. A child who senses that adults cannot listen to what they say about this will soon learn to suppress it and be left with sensory impressions that have not been processed verbally. This processing eases the integration of these impressions into long-term memory, and reduces the likelihood of PTSD.

Early help

Following the immediate phase, one should be careful about forcing an emotional-processing of the event on the child. Let children do this at their own pace, but be aware of their signals and check with them whether they are harbouring fantasies or are experiencing intrusive images or thoughts about what happened. Children's capacity to regulate their emotions develops gradually and they often avoid long conversations about something that is painful. If they do not want to talk, there may be several reasons for this; for example, it is too painful, they do not feel the need, they are afraid of not being understood, they feel guilty, etc. Be patient, do not pressurize them to talk but be ready to follow up on their cues. If the child seems to be doing well in school and does not start to isolate him/herself and the child's behaviour does not undergo serious changes, there are usually no reasons for concern.

'First Aid Tips'

- Go through what happened to make sure that the child (and family) have an overview and understanding;
- Follow up on thoughts the children experienced when they learned about what happened and afterwards;
- If the child has taken in strong sensory impressions or has created strong fantasies based on what happened, e.g., observing a father shoot himself, let him/her express these in words or drawings. Provide him/her with simple self-help strategies to take control of these (see Stallard 2002);
- Ask about the reactions the child experienced when he/she learnt about what happened and afterwards. Sensitively describe normal reactions in order for him/her to be able to recognize them, if they experience them. Be sure to say that he/she does not *have* to experience this to be normal, but that these reactions are what other children who have lost someone close have described;
- Stimulate expression of thoughts and emotions through play, art activities and rituals, and help the child develop a 'narrative' or story about what they have experienced;
- If new facts about the death become known, inform the child;
- Give the child suggestions about what others have done that has helped them, including talking with friends, advice about sleep, etc.;
- Advise adult caregivers on how they can create stability in children's life and how to make contact for further help;
- Encourage contact with friends and help children think about how to explain what has happened to them.

Sometimes the family's reactions to a death by suicide may necessitate meetings with professionals or volunteers to facilitate or restore family communication. Provide the family with advice on how to access bereavement services and encourage them to talk to their family doctor.

Many children have good coping resources and will make good use of self-care strategies. However, a death by suicide is a powerful event that can be difficult to manage over time for many children.

Early therapeutic help may help in preventing unnecessary long-term problems and newer methods developed for complicated grief and post-traumatic stress problems may benefit children. Although resources are scarce, it is important to try to refer children sooner rather than later. Some guidelines about when to refer are found in Cohen *et al.* (2002). In all therapy, it will be important to restore children's experience of control and predictability in their life.

In addition to the psycho-educative and supportive efforts aimed at the individual child, it is very important that the child bereaved by suicide is included in family communication about the suicide. Through open, honest, and direct communication about facts, and feelings about what happened, the child will be able to integrate the suicide as they go through the developmental phases in childhood and adolescence. It is important that children are given age-related support and help, and that the principles for help are applied at home, at school, or in the nursery. Further information on advice concerning bereaved children can be found in Dyregrov (1991).

Help for the family bereaved by suicide

Work to help the family starts on the day of the suicide. The main aim is to ensure that family members are carefully looked after, and to start normalizing the situation in cooperation with the bereaved family. By reducing distress, and re-establishing a kind of order and structure, the individual and the family can be helped to restore function and 'a normal life'. It is very important that helpers map the aspects of the actual situation and encourage the individual and the family's strength and coping resources.

Emotional 'first aid' may be given at a hospital, by the ambulance personnel, the clergyman, crisis teams, or by local community health support workers. The bereaved should be met with calmness, support, and empathy, in a situation that is chaotic and unreal. Psychoeducative information should be provided for the bereaved from the day of the suicide, and repeated over time. On the first day, the capacity for taking in such information is often limited. More information about common psychological or psychosocial difficulties or reactions that they may experience can be provided after some days and may need repetition.

To be able to comprehend and start re-constructing a world that has fallen apart, information about the death is essential. It is important to help family members access information to order, and structure what happened.

Within a couple of days after the suicide, it may be appropriate to provide the family with more information. Initial advice and written information for the family are of utmost importance in contributing to the initiation of the grief process and to normalizing and possibly reducing traumatic reactions. It is important that guidance be provided early in order for parents to make decisions about whether children should see the deceased. Advice about when belongings of the deceased should be removed should also be provided early on, before well meaning friends and relatives start clearing things away too fast. Information about the importance of participation in rituals and the importance of including children in these should be provided. It is also important to give information about the inquest, post-mortem and other legal events that will take place during the first days following the death. It is important, in a sensitive manner, to prepare the bereaved for the existential crisis that many will experience with its ensuing trauma, crisis, and grief reactions. Later on, gender differences, problems related to family dynamics, children's reactions, and the way grief changes over time, should be stressed. However, professionals should not present these aspects in such a manner that people may feel there is something wrong with them if they do not encounter such problems. The timing, as well as the quantity and the quality of the information, must be attuned to the needs of the individual or family. Information, and other kinds of intervention, must be related to the specific situation, as experienced by the individual family affected by the suicide.

Ideally, every family bereaved by suicide should be offered the opportunity to meet with a grief counsellor to discuss family communication, the children's reactions and behaviour, and family dynamics. The frequency of the meetings should be adjusted to the needs of the individual family, but aim at contact close to memorial days (dates of birth and death) and major holidays. Counselling may include individual advice on the necessity of returning to painful places or activities, and discussion of common reactions connected to the birthday and death-day of the deceased. It is important to advise parents as to how to care for bereaved children, as well as to support and encourage their successful efforts. The bereaved need information about available psychosocial health care provision and how they may apply for additional help.

Prepare the family for situations and circumstances that they will encounter as time goes on (e.g. gender differences in grief, reactions of others, etc.). Because of the frequent disturbance of memory function in the wake of a traumatic loss, it is helpful to provide information both orally and in written form.

Helping agencies need to acknowledge that some families lack or have very restricted or unhelpful social networks, so that effort may be required to mobilize these. Professionals and volunteers can prepare the bereaved family for other people's often disappointing or hurtful reactions, and give advice on how to manage this. Finally, information about, and offers to attend support groups or NGO-support organizations may be provided through distribution of leaflets. Information about support groups such as 'Survivors of Bereavement by Suicide' (UK) can be very useful.

Conclusion

A suicide in the family is a devastating experience for the adults and children left behind; often resulting in a tremendous and long lasting impact. Besides the individual suffering of family members, the family's communication and structure is also tested. Bereaved people ask for help from both professionals and social networks. They want immediate and outreach help from trained personnel, they seek information, various kinds of assistance, more help for children, the opportunity to meet with others who have been bereaved, and help provided over time. In order to secure adequate help for *all* families bereaved by suicide, routine community intervention programmes should be implemented. Based on the experience of the bereaved in our nationwide studies in Norway, we have presented some principles for crisis and bereavement intervention.

Although we have outlined a philosophy of caring and a strategy for help, we wish to stress that every family is unique. Every individual and every family should be met and helped on the basis of *their* needs. The challenge for social network members and professionals alike is to withhold our own concepts about what families are experiencing and what help we think they need, and listen carefully to what they tell us.

References

Cohen JA, Mannarino AP, Greenberg T *et al.* (2002). Childhood traumatic grief. *Trauma, Violence, and Abuse* **3**:307–27.

Dyregrov A (1991). *Grief in children. A handbook for adults.* London: Jessica Kingsley.

Dyregrov A (1996). Children's participation in rituals. *Bereavement Care* **15**:2–5.

Dyregrov K (2001). Søsken etter selvmord. In: A Dyregrov, G Lorentzen, and K Raaheim (ed.), *Et liv for barn. Utfordringer, omsorg og hjelpetiltak,* (s.146–58). Bergen: Fagbokforlaget.

Dyregrov K (2002). Assistance from local authorities versus survivors' needs for support after suicide. *Death Studies* **26**:647–69.

Dyregrov K (2003). *The loss of a child by suicide, SIDS, and accidents; consequences, needs and provision of help.* Doctoral Dissertation (Dr. Philos), Faculty of Psychology, HEMIL - University of Bergen, Bergen, Norway.

Dyregrov K, Nordanger D, Dyregrov A (2003). Predictors of psychosocial distress after suicide, SIDS, and accidents. *Death Studies* **27**:143–65.

Janoff-Bulman R (1992). *Shattered assumptions. Towards a new psychology of trauma.* New York: The Free Press.

Li X, Precht DH, Mortensen PB *et al.* (2003). Mortality in parents after death of a child in Denmark: a nationwide follow-up study. *The Lancet* **361**, 363–7.

Murphy SA (2000). The use of research findings in bereavement programs: a case study. *Death Studies* **24**:585–602.

Neimeyer RA (2000). Searching for the meaning of meaning: grief therapy and the process of reconstruction. *Death Studies* **24**:541–58.

Oliver L (1999). Effects of a child's death on the marital relationship: a review. *Omega –Journal of Death and Dying* **39**:197–227.

Parkes CM (1998). Coping with loss: bereavement in adult life. *British Medical Journal* **316**:856–9.

Pfeffer CR, Martins P, Mann J *et al.* (1997). Child survivors of suicide: psychosocial characteristics. *Journal of American Academy of Child and Adolescent Psychiatry* **36**:1, 65–74.

Prigerson HG, Shear MK, Jacobs SC *et al.* (2000). Grief and its relation to PTSD. In: D Nutt, Jr T Davidson (ed.), *Post traumatic stress disorders: diagnosis, management and treatment* pp. 163–86. New York: Martin Dunitz.

Provini C, Everett JR, Pfeffer CR (2000). Adults mourning suicide: self-reported concerns about bereavement, needs for assistance, and help-seeking behavior. *Death Studies* **24**:1–9.

Rakic AS (1992). *Sibling survivors of adolescent suicide.* Dissertation Doctor of Philosophy, The California School of Professional Psychology Berkeley/Alameda.

Raundalen M (2000). Hva skal vi si til barn om selvmord? *Suicidologi* **5**:12–15.

Schwab R (1998). A child's death and divorce: dispelling the myth. *Death Studies* **22**:445–68.

Stallard P (2002). *Think good – feel good. a cognitive behaviour therapy workbook for children and young people.* Chichester: John Wiley & Sons Ltd.

Survivors of Bereavement by Suicide (UK) www.uk-sobs.org.uk

Chapter 15

Family liaison: when once has to be enough

Julie Ellison

What is Family Liaison?

The newspapers report tragedy all the time; murders, rapes, traffic collisions, and frequently the report is followed by the words, 'Police family liaison officers are comforting the family'.

So, who are these family liaison officers, and what do they do?

Family Liaison has always been a function of the police, although for many years, it was generally confined to homicide enquiries. A police officer was assigned to liaise with the bereaved family and keep them informed about the investigation. For most families, it is important to know how the police are progressing with enquiries into the death of their loved ones. For some, the grieving process cannot even begin to start, until they know that the person responsible for killing their loved one has been apprehended and a sentence passed upon them. The role of the Family Liaison Officer is to update them at regular intervals and inform them of the progress in their investigation. Officers asked to perform this role received no training and did not know what was required of them. Rarely did two officers operate in the same way and there were no guidelines to help them. The assignment was not much sought after, yet, despite this set back, feedback from the families was frequently good. Officers realised they were dealing with traumatized bereaved family members from a variety of cultures, who had little, or no experience of the judicial system, and they tried their best to help them, despite the lack of training or support. They tried to deliver news with as much compassion and sensitivity as possible and many families felt that they did this well—but other families did not feel that they received any satisfactory service. The difficulties of the role were highlighted during the investigation into the murder of Stephen Lawrence.

Stephen was an 18-year-old black student. In 1993, he and a friend of his were travelling home and were attacked by a group of youths. Stephen was stabbed and died at the scene. The resulting police investigation was strongly criticized by Stephen's family, and there were several reviews of police procedure. A public Inquiry was set up in 1999, which was conducted by Sir William Macpherson. Much of the Inquiry focused on the way that family liaison had been managed.

The Inquiry reported that:

> From the first contact with police officers at the hospital and thereafter, Mr and Mrs Lawrence were treated with insensitivity and lack of sympathy. One of the saddest and most deplorable aspects of the case concerns the failure of Family Liaison. Mr and Mrs Lawrence were not dealt with or treated as they should have been. They were patronized. They were never given information about the investigation to which they were entitled. Family Liaison failed, despite the good intentions of the officers allocated to this task. Senior officers never intervened to rectify the failure (Macpherson 1999).

The Inquiry team made more than 70 recommendations; several that concerned Family Liaison. They stated that (Macpherson 1999):

- Police services should ensure that at local level there are readily available designated and trained Family Liaison Officers

- Training of Family Liaison Officers must include training in racism awareness and cultural diversity, so that families are treated appropriately, professionally, with respect and according to their needs

- Family Liaison Officers shall, where appointed, be dedicated primarily if not exclusively to that task

- Senior Investigating Officers and Family Liaison Officers be made aware that good practice and their positive duty shall be the satisfactory management of family liaison, together with the provision to a victim's family of all possible information about the crime and its investigation

- Good practice shall provide that any request made by the family of a victim that is not acceded to, and any complaint by any member of the family, shall be formally recorded by the SIO and shall be reported to the immediate superior officer

- Police Services and Victim Support Services ensure that their systems provide for the pro-active use of local contacts within the minority ethnic communities to assist family liaison where appropriate.

It was a difficult period for the Metropolitan Police Service, but it also provided an opportunity to review and to learn. Some progress had already been made by the time the MacPherson Report was published, and some training had already been started with the support of other forces. All police forces in the United Kingdom provided some form of Family Liaison training for their own officers.

Training for Family Liaison Officers was planned by the Metropolitan Police Service department responsible for FLOs at Scotland Yard, the Detective Training School (now the Crime Academy) at Hendon and representatives from voluntary and statuatory organizations.

At the time of writing, over 850 MPS Officers have been trained on the Family Liaison course. The Crime Academy at Hendon Police Training College runs an FLO Course for 16 students every three weeks, see Fig. 15.1.

The course lasts 6 days and deals with the various issues a bereaved family may encounter and with which an FLO may have to help. All teaching is conducted in a small group setting, with exercises and group discussions.

	CRIME ACADEMY of NEW SCOTLAND YARD **FAMILY LIAISON OFFICERS COURSE**
TIMETABLE	
Sunday	**Introduction and Administration** **Family Liaison History**—McPherson recommendations 23–28 **What is a family**—Circle exercise
Monday	**The Role of the FLO**—Exercise and definition **First Contact and the FLO Log**—Accountability and best practice **The Identification Process**—How we can help families with this at the mortuary **FLO Strategy & Tactics**—Disclosure of information, how the FLO works with the family, split families, suspects within the family. Definitions, discussion and exercise around minimum standards
Tuesday	**Bereavements in Adults, Children and Families**—Candle Project: Covers Sudden and Traumatic Death and the FLO's role
Wednesday	**The Role of the Coroner**—Visiting speaker is usually a Coroners Officer **The Criminal Justice System**—All aspects up to the Appeal Court. Also Civil cases and private prosecutions **Victimology**—Obtaining information and intelligence about the victim **Cross Border Family Liaison**—FLOs from different Police Service areas, here and overseas **Victim Support**—Visiting speaker from Victim Support. Role of other outside agencies
Thursday	**Visiting Speaker from the Diversity Directorate, New Scotland Yard**—The role of this team, also covers exit strategies and mass disaster plans **Independent Advice**—The role of the Independent Advisory Groups in the Metropolitan Police Service **The Law of Homicide and the Road Traffic Act**—The difference between murder and death by dangerous driving–questions and discussion **Achieving Best Evidence**—ABE—Use of video interviews etc. for vulnerable witnesses
Friday	**Occupational Health**—Outside speaker from O.H., self-monitoring of stress and referral to O.H. **Scenarios**—Dilemmas for discussion in groups **Course Debrief** **Closure and Evaluation**—This course is always closed by a senior officer from the Diversity Directorate at New Scotland Yard

Reproduced by kind permission of DC Ron Cuthbertson, Crime Academy

Fig. 15.1

The Involvement of the Candle Project

The Candle Project was first involved with Metropolitan Police Service Family Liaison following the Ladbroke Grove Rail Crash in 1999. Large numbers of FLOs were deployed as there were a large number of casualties—31 fatalities and hundreds injured. Some of the bereaved included families with young children. FLOs were being asked by families as to how they could break the news to children and how to deal with their responses. Expert help was needed to ensure that the needs of the children were met with. The Candle Project at St Christopher's Hospice was able to give professional advice to the FLOs during that time and provide copies of their booklet 'Someone Has Died Suddenly' (1999), to officers working with families.

The team planning the FLO Training involved Candle from the outset, as part of a group of interested professionals and volunteers from the bereavement field.

Who can become an FLO?

Sir Ian Blair, Deputy Commissioner of the Metropolitan Police states that, 'The loss of a close family member or friend through sudden, violent or unexplained death, is one of the most traumatic experiences. Inevitably, the police service becomes involved in such events and family liaison plays a fundamental part in the investigation of such deaths. The importance of Family Liaison is enormous. The interaction with a bereaved family can be critical to the success or failure of investigations and therefore the skills of Family Liaison Officers (FLOs) are vital tools for investigation managers.' (*Association of Chief Police Officers 2003.*)

Any officer may apply to be an FLO, but they must make written application to their line manager outlining the skills and qualities they have that might make them suitable for the role. Their application must be supported by their line manager before being passed on to the FLO Team at New Scotland Yard. Officers are asked to provide details, not just about their policing skills, but also about their background and religion. If they speak another language, this is also noted. These details enable them to be matched to a family, in case a Senior Investigating Officer in an Inquiry request an officer with particular skills or experience.

Officers are expected to be experienced interviewers and investigators – the primary role of an FLO is that of an investigator. They need to be able to elicit information from families or friends at a time when the victims are probably traumatized.

This may sound harsh—it might seem that all the family might need at this time would be compassion and empathy. Certainly, Family Liaison Officers are expected to be compassionate, but they need to be capable of much more. Families also want justice and the key to an investigation may lie in the detailed information that only the family can provide.

In a murder investigation, where there are no initial leads to the motive or suspect, information from friends or those close to the victim, can prove to be vital. Information such as why the victim was in a particular place at a particular time, their routines, hobbies, and habits is what is known as 'victimology.' FLOs know that this information is of vital importance – if you can find out how a victim lived, you may very well find out how they died.

The stresses on officers who become very close to the families they work with, are appreciated by the Metropolitan Police Service, and a system of welfare support has been established. All applicants are vetted by the MPS's Occupational Health Directorate and their sickness record examined. They are then expected to complete a questionnaire to provide further information about their personal history and any other life events. Many officers are also called for individual interviews. In most cases, an officer who has experienced a bereavement, divorce, or serious illness within the previous 18 months is asked to delay their application.

First Contact: Breaking Bad News

Many bereaved families say that the most traumatic moment in their lives was the notification of the death of their loved one. Those people who have been asked to inform someone about the death of their partner, child, spouse, sibling, or friend find this the most difficult and stressful part of their job.

Although most Police Forces try to choose a trained FLO to break the bad news to a family, this is not always possible. Many forces do not have large numbers of trained FLOs and a trained officer is not always on duty at the time a death-message needs to be delivered. Sensitive news needs to be delivered as soon as possible, but it is important to try to establish key areas of information before speaking to the family.

The following extract is taken from 'Breaking Bad News' (A Practical Guide for Delivering Death Messages to Families) Metropolitan Police Service Publication 2003: (Fig. 15.2).

Experience suggests that the family will usually want to know all available details of the incident. It is important that the officer is primed with this information, as far as possible, before speaking to the family. However, breaking news is often reported on the television even before the police have been informed of the incident. In this instance, it may not be possible to gather as much information, as one would want before going to speak to the family. The dilemma is whether to wait until sufficient information has been gathered, or to go anyway. Any delay allows someone else with even less information to inform the family. A formal source of information, such as the police, is preferred while breaking bad news. The police have some training and are able to contain the situation for the bereaved family.

There is no easy way to break the news of a death to a family, particularly if the death has happened suddenly and the family has had no preparation for it. Very often, they are shocked and do not believe the news. They are unable to take in all the information, especially, if the death is a result of murder. The police officer relaying the news, or the Family Liaison Officer, may have to repeat the information several times. If there is a criminal investigation into the death, delays may occur before viewing the body is possible and funeral arrangements can be made, so that forensic evidence can be collected. Frequently, the body may be disfigured, if the death was violent or involved a severe traumatic impact. All these things can be difficult to explain to a family, especially if children are involved.

Delivering bad news when children are present

When a Family Liaison Officer goes to an address to deliver a death message, they will have the name of the next of kin, but probably not much more than that. Sometimes, there will be other adults and children in the house. The arrival of a police officer at the door will herald bad news for many adults. The fear is already there as soon as the

BREAKING BAD NEWS

Prior to delivering the death message, the following points need to be considered:-

- Establish that we are delivering the right message to the right person.
- Know where the victim is at the time of delivering the message so the family can go there if they wish.
- Attempt to establish if there will be any communication requirements as regards language or disability.
- Attempt to find out as much as you are able to about the circumstances of the incident to tell the family.
- Do not assume that a neighbour is the best person to help the family or be with them when giving the message. If we choose a neighbour it may not be a person that the family either know or like.
- Be prepared to face new emotion.

However, none of the above should delay us in delivering the message if there is a chance of the family finding out from any other source. We must be the ones to tell them first.

What to do

- If the officer is in plain clothes they must clearly identify themselves and ask to enter the premises.
- If the officer is in uniform ask to enter the premises.
  Ask the person or people that we are about to give the message, to sit down.

What to say

- I am very sorry to tell you that **use name** (meaning – use the name of the dead person) is dead or has been killed.
- I am afraid that I have very bad news. **Use name** is dead or has been killed.
- If the first contact is to be held in the family home, wait until you are asked to be seated, as sitting in the wrong chair, i.e. the one the dead person always sat in can upset the family. If the first contact is at your workplace, ensure there are sufficient seats and the family are allowed to sit where they wish especially if they have brought someone along to support them.
- Ask the family how they wish you to refer to them. It is often better to start off on the more formal basis i.e. Mr or Mrs.
- Ask the family how they wish you to refer to the victim.
- Don't say **'Are you happy with that'** – the word happy and the bereaved do not go together.
- Don't try to finish family members sentences for them. Bereaved people will take time to formulate what they want to say to you.

Fig. 15.2 Taken from 'Breaking Bad News (A Practical Guide for Delivering Death Messages to Families)' (2003), Metropolitan Police Service Publication.

door is opened. A child may react very differently. Their natural curiosity will be aroused, especially if the officer is in uniform. This presents a dilemma for the officer, who has to decide very quickly, whether to go ahead with the message, or to ask for the child to leave the room. Too often, children are the forgotten victims in the death of a family member. We know they are there, but how do we begin to explain to them the death of a person who is probably very special to them? The adults are often so bewildered and shocked that they are unable to help their children. However the news is delivered, the family will never forget the details of that moment. There is no second chance to make a first impression.

The FLO's training has helped them prepare themselves for such situations. The family will probably look to them for advice. Some families may even ask the FLO to tell the child the news on their behalf, as they cannot face doing so themselves. The FLO will normally try to enable the parent to do this, as it is important not to dis-empower them. The police officer is only a transitory presence in this family's life. The surviving parent will be there in the long days ahead, when the child feels ready to ask the difficult questions. It will be of no use to them if the only person prepared to give them answers, is the police officer who is no longer there.

Sometimes once has to be enough

The following case examples from FLOs illustrate the work that can be done during one visit following the above guidelines. Though often we have only one meeting with a family and our first responsibility is towards the investigation, yet much can be achieved.

Case Example 1

An officer from the Traffic Division was asked to break the news to a woman that her husband had died in a fatal crash with his motorbike, while on his way to work. The officer found her at home alone and broke the news. The woman, Mrs F, was very distressed and broke off in the middle of her tears to tell the officer that her six year old son was coming home in ten minutes from school. She didn't feel able to tell him the news. Could he do it?

The officer talked to Mrs F, reassuring her that he would not leave her alone and that if necessary he would start the conversation with her son. He pointed out to her gently that as soon as he reached home, her son would know that something was wrong when he saw her so upset, with a stranger. Did she really want her son to hear such important news from a stranger rather than his mother?

Eventually, Mrs F was able to tell her child the news, with the help of the officer. He stayed with her until other family members arrived, supported her through her child's first reactions and made an arrangement to come back to answer any questions they might have, a few days later. At the meeting, he undertook to find the mirror from Mr F's motorbike, which had been undamaged in the crash and to return it to his son, who had specifically requested something to remember his father by.

Case Example 2

Mr and Mrs G's son, Robert, aged 14, had been killed on his way home from school after being involved in a fight with some other youths. The parents focused on the search for justice and would not allow any support agency's access to them or to their other son, John. They did not believe that counselling would help them.

The FLO was the only professional who was in contact with them when the case against the young men came to trial. Although they were found guilty, the sentences felt very inadequate to the G's as punishment for the death of their son. The FLO was able to persuade them to make contact with SAMM (Support After Murder and Manslaughter) and a bereavement project for children, to give them an opportunity to talk this through.

Case Example 3

Mrs N and her husband lived in a flat with their four young children, two boys and a girl under the age of six and Jamie, their 8 month-old son. Mrs N's husband left for work early in the morning and the children went to join their mother for a cuddle in bed, as she dozed off, on account of a late-night-feed for Jamie.

Mrs N, who must have fallen asleep, woke up to feel her feet were hot and realized with shock that the duvet and the bottom of the bed were on fire. She managed to grab hold of the older children and drag them outside. She then attempted to go back into the house to rescue Jamie, who was in his cot beside the bed. Unfortunately, she was beaten back by the flames and neighbours had to forcibly restrain her from trying to get back in.

The Fire Brigade managed to rescue Jamie, but he died in hospital shortly afterwards from burns and smoke inhalation.

Family Liaison Officers were involved from the outset. They provided support to the family at the hospital and helped the medical staff break the news of Jamie's death to the other relatives arriving at the hospital. Early investigations revealed that the likely cause of the fire was the duvet being set on fire by a cigarette lighter. The parents confirmed that the two boys had been told off recently for lighting matches and had developed a fascination flames. It seemed they might have started the fire that had killed their brother.

Despite their own grief, the parents were anxious to avoid any sense of guilt or blame being attached to their sons, and were keen to ensure they did everything possible to ease the pain of their surviving children. Working together with the Coroner's Officer, and having sought advice from the Candle Project, the FLOs discussed the possibility of the children seeing their brother. The parents were not adverse to this, but were unsure how best to do it. They were worried that the children might be distressed by the sight of their brother, who had burns to his face.

The children were asked to bring a toy for their brother. The FLOs and the Coroner's Officer spoke to them first together with their parents. They were told that Jamie would look as if he were sleeping, but that he was not asleep, because his body would not work any more. He had been too little to cope with the very hot fire and smoke and so had died. He would not be able to speak or play with them any more, and his body would now feel very cold.

Case Example 3—cont'd

They were also told that his face and hands had red marks on it from the fire. The children were led into the room by their parents, accompanied by the FLOs, and the Coroner's Officer. The parents lifted them up to see their baby brother and invited them to give him the toys they had brought for him, so that he would not look so lonely. The children were fascinated by their brother. They were interested in his burns and were allowed to touch and kiss him.

It was an emotional moment for all involved but proved to be a vitally important part in the investigation, as one of the boys told Jamie that he was sorry for having started the fire. He was immediately hugged by his parents and told that they did not blame him but loved him, although they were very sad that Jamie had died.

The three children later had to be interviewed on video for the purposes of the Coroner's Inquest by the Family Liaison Officers. All the family were referred to the Traumatic Stress Clinic at the Maudsley Hospital in London. The children attended the funeral and all drew pictures for their brother which they placed on his tiny coffin, along with flowers.

Current state of play and future

The Family Liaison Team at New Scotland Yard oversees all matters concerned with Family Liaison and is responsible for all connected projects. They also are responsible for forging links with partner agencies and provide a training facility for both police and outside agencies. They act as Advisors for anyone, including FLOs and Co-ordinators, who requires assistance about a Family Liaison issue.

The unit has a close working relationship with the Foreign and Commonwealth Office, as well as the Anti-Terrorist Branch. Family Liaison Officers have previously been assigned to the families of victims who died in the World Trade Centre, Bali and Istanbul bombings. They will play a vital role in any future mass disasters.

A video entitled 'The Message', designed to give an awareness of the effect of the death upon a family and provide guidance on liaison with them, has recently been released (2003). It is aimed at all police employees who may have contact with the bereaved. The film shows seven bereaved families talking about their experiences of the delivery of the death-message and the impact of the subsequent investigation. It was designed with the help of many victim's families and support organizations, and includes the recommendations made in the Stephen Lawrence Inquiry (1999) and the public Inquiry into The Identification of Victims Following Major Transport Accidents (March 2001). In the words of Lord Justice Clark, who conducted the latter Inquiry, 'Respect for the dead and for the relatives of those who have died, especially where the death has been unexpected, is indeed the mark of a civilized society'.

Conclusion

FLOs are not counsellors. If there is a need for the help and support of a counsellor or any other special support, FLOs can help to make arrangements, quickly and confidentially, to put families in touch with agencies with experience in this area.

We recognize that there are distinct limitations in what can be done when one or two contacts are all we may have. Experience has taught us, however, to appreciate the importance of these contacts. Families bereaved by a sudden death are often greatly shocked and traumatized. They look to the police officer for reassurance and reliability, in a world that has become very unsafe and insecure. What we do, however short term, can make a very real difference.

References

Breaking bad news (a practical guide for delivering death messages to families) (2003). London: A Metropolitan Police Service Publication.

Family liaison policy and fundamental guidelines (2001). London: A Metropolitan Police Service Publication.

Family liaison strategy manual (2003). London: Association of Chief Police Officers Publication.

Macpherson W (1999). *The Stephen Lawrence Inquiry.* London: HMSO.

Public inquiry into the identification of victims following major transport accidents (2001). London: HMSO.

Candle (1999). *Someone has died suddenly.* London: St Christopher's Hospice.

The message (2003). London: A Metropolitan Police Service Publication.

Chapter 16

Crossing the great barrier grief

Stewart Sinclair

Introduction and history

Blue mood rising

Two blue tanagers (common birds in this part of the Caribbean) court and make love in the wisps of the Casuarina tree, as the early morning sun disperses the steamy secrets of the tropical night. As the light increases, noisy little nocturnal tree frogs have gone quiet and the contented couple of tanagers sing post-coital melodies to the dawn of the new day.

I am looking towards the horizon, from my hotel balcony at that indeterminate point of uncertain reality, where the blue sky of this tropic meets the blue sea, and I think back to those happy distant days when Susan and I scraped our wages together to elevate youthful love from campsites in Margate, in the back of a very ancient Land Rover, to the sensory delights of a world where the vision captured by Kew Gardens in a London bubble is liberated; and perhaps where the glass-framed plants of Decimus Burton's palace secretly dream about in their leafy slumbers in the long grey English winter.

I am at the end of my holiday in this blue world, and it has been nine years since Susan died of breast cancer, and my two boys—Thomas now aged 16 and James aged 13—are asleep in the next room. Thomas is no doubt sleeping off his Carib beer-hangover and James yearns to be old enough to have his own hangover, but substitutes this age deficit by overdosing on spaghetti bolognese, instead.

The tranquillity of this moment is, of course, illusory. At holiday time, we escape from our own daily struggles, if we can, to lands where for two weeks, we do not want to hear about other countries' hurricanes, poverty, and problems, when we are on the run from our own.

For many parents who have lost their partner, holidays can be a critical point in the adjustment/recovery process, where the jumble of thoughts and emotions of guilt, sadness, and loss are on collision course with that mysterious and indeterminate horizon point, where they hit the brutal realities of the present and the primitive and complex tasks of rescuing the ability of enjoyment and love from an ocean of grief and tragedy.

In my blue holiday world, the colour of my mood is not blue; the blue tanagers have made love and the blues of the sky flirt mischievously and are tickled by the waving palm fronds, and nearly ripe mangoes dangle seductively from their green iridescent canopy, all paying homage to the timeless healing alchemy of nature, and its ability, and capacity to navigate the fragilities of life, and rebuild, and reconstruct, and regrow, even if the hurricane is personal or regional.

Just as the mariners of old did not fall off the edge of their world at that illusive and elusive horizon point, neither have I slipped over that fearfully real but metaphorical edge, despite having the conventional bearings and reference points of life being ripped away from myself and Thomas and James, by the death of Susan; losing her to that sordid and malignant destiny of mutating cells.

We are all still here, though, the three of us; perhaps more aware of the frailty of life than the majority of people in the affluent world. My children laugh and play like other children; and it still hurts me when I hear those other children shout 'mum' on the beach – but somehow we are all here, not just in body, but in spirit, as well. Our pathway is, of course, different because we all realized that Susan's death shattered ordinariness and orderliness and we instantly knew that that world was gone forever.

Desolate, devastated, and adrift in this post-Susan world where reference points and charts and constellations were meaningless markers of the past, the prolonged assistance our family received from our local hospice, and the personal help I received from the Dimbleby Cancer Care Centre, also for a very prolonged period, were priceless contributors in assisting the three of us to establish and chart a new life course that has included an holistic combination of practical interventions and a less easy-to-define injection of soul chemistry that has led to post-Susan secular, but nonetheless spiritual resurrection and what I like to think is a vigorous grip on life.

The professional help, channelled to our family cannot be overstated regarding the positive impact it has had prior to, and following the death of Susan, who was without doubt, at the very least the captain of our ship, and at the most a kind and thoughtful and gentle person; only occasionally forced to become a Dominatrix, when mutiny was threatened by her motley crew, which included me—a most reluctant father. As her physical health waned, and with the help of Hospice support, and family and friends, Susan supervised the smooth transfer from the rank of a captain to that of a reluctant seafarer.

The professional and informal help received was in the aspect of the 'transfer'—a crucial aspect in helping to retain and relocate so many of Susan's strengths into our new world, and even to this day and a new career, it is not grief and sadness that reign when thinking of Susan, but it is the thoughts of her as a driving force of our recovery and the passing on of a spiritual inheritance of her enthusiasm for life, that is constant and undimmed by death, and still lights the smiles of Thomas and James, as they—motherless—chart their own courses in life, enveloped by a powerful unconscious sense of their own history and self.

With so much help received from our local hospice, contact with others in similar predicaments to my own was natural and inevitable and through professional and user contacts, it soon became apparent that there was a very significant gap in service provision for those who are parents of young and teenaged children, who have lost partners.

Indeed, one of the things that I had highlighted to those helping our family was the absence of a self-help support group, and subsequently Angela Paul and myself were asked to assist St Christopher's Hospice to help them establish a parent/carers group.

Angela is a young African-Caribbean mother of St Lucian descent with two young children at the time of her husband, Sean's death, from skin cancer in St Christopher's Hospice. Like my own family, they had all received much assistance from the local Hospice and Angela had also noticed the same gap in service for the bereaved parent, at a time when a deluge of sympathy, empathy, and offers were being poured onto our children.

Angela and I were then asked to become the advisory and steering group members of the St Christopher's Candle Project and from there on the embryonic ideas for developing the group became a reality and the Parents and Carers have now been meeting for nearly four years, after having had our first meeting in November 1999. Angela and I have completely different social and professional backgrounds (which will be referred to later), but either by design or good fortune, this combination seems to have worked in attracting and holding a hugely diverse collection of attenders together. In part, this is due to the astonishing resourcefulness of Angela (who is the only person I have ever known) who can lose a passport on Saturday morning, replace it the same morning at the Passport Office, and still catch a flight at Heathrow Airport by lunchtime to attend a Palliative Care conference in Sicily to talk about our group.

Important components of the practical structure such as child care and transport

When bereavement overwhelms a family, sometimes the daily practicalities of life fragment along different fault-lines. If you do not have a motor car and you do not have easy access to professional or extended family child care help, or when you are suddenly on your own—with a child or children—many things, that had been taken for granted as part of a shared relationship, are shattered. Even at the bus or train station, how do you go to the toilet, when you have a child or children and baggage? You no longer have a partner to help you with the pushchair on the bus or coach, and you have to rely on a public who may or may not be inclined to assist. Of course, single parents are familiar with these situations, but those who find themselves in this predicament through the death of a partner are not, and the psychological dis-ablement can at times be enduring and profound, and can generate unexpected stress and sadness, and despair, when you are perhaps tired and waiting for a train that is endlessly delayed and the bags very heavy, and the children crying, and it is cold and raining.

All these things are real pressures to some bereaved parents; to others, the fault-lines might have different consequences. At the Candle Project meetings, we thought through as many of these issues as possible prior to establishing the group, to see where best we might be able to use our limited resources to make our group as available as possible to everyone, no matter what their social class and resource situation might be.

With the help of volunteers who had been trained and selected and Criminal Records Bureau checked, we were in a position to provide safe and reliable transport for those who needed it to attend each meeting; and at the meeting of the group itself, all the children could be looked after by the volunteers. The 'looking after' is not just 'minding'; it is actively involving the children in various stimulating games and crafts and it encompasses an age range from baby to teenager.

As noted above, the 'fall-out' is different for all of us, but the universal theme that emerged in planning and setting up the group was the crucial need to have the time and the space away from our children, but in the knowledge and comfort that they were nearby, in an environment with safe and secure child-care. Through the dedication and reliability of these volunteers, the group has achieved a very important objective for bereaved parents. It has created a brief, but regular protective capsule of time and space, where we can share our experiences of grief and simultaneously assist each other in the recovery and adjustment process. Sometimes it is grim; sometimes it is funny, and sometimes it just cannot be captured in words, but the eloquence of unwritten and sometimes unspoken sadness forms a strange alchemy that can only be found in a self-help group.

The logistics of managing our group can be seen as daunting, especially, when others are thinking of developing such a service in their own area from nothing; however, they are obviously surpassable or else, we would not be there. Our available resources allow us to have three meetings a year with full child care support, and we have a number of other meetings such as summer outings, Christmas gatherings, for instance, where we either bring our children, or make our own child-care arrangements.

To summarize what we have identified, the most important aspects of our Parent/Carer group are as follows:

◆ transport resources to take members home as well as collecting them and a place to meet;

◆ excellent child-care services to allow time and space away from our children;

◆ feeling safe;

◆ being comfortable if you are not articulate and being comfortable if you are;

◆ feeling safe, whether you are a man or woman;

◆ feeling you are in the right place irrespective of your religious or cultural or ethnic background;

◆ helping to ease the sadness of isolation post-bereavement;

◆ helping to assess the natural context of sadness and depression by using the group to help and monitor ourselves in a safe and informal environment. When it is not normal, we can help one another to seek out the appropriate assistance;

◆ Using group leaders, or however you define such entities, who, if at all possible balance gender and ethnicity.

Operating a subtle and gentle hierarchy within a user control/self-help philosophy

An important feature of the group is obviously its informality and its social context, although there are boundaries which will be noted later in this chapter. My own professional expertise is in the area of health and social care, and Angela has a professional background in the commercial sector. It is by chance that I have experience in managing groups, and in managing the dynamics that groups always generate and this has sat comfortably with Angela's perspective of the group process.

We were neither 'elected', nor do we serve a set term of office, and the boundaries of democracy may be a little blurred, but then this is often the nature of self-help groups where 'product champions' as they would be called in the business world, set out to establish an innovative design, product, or service.

To counterbalance any tendency to autocracy, or over-controlling attitudes, or indeed any attitude problems at all, there is a supervisory and accountability framework. Both Angela and I report to and are supervised by and accountable to the Project Leader at the Candle Project. Clearly, the Parent/Carer Group is an informal but structured partnership with the Hospice, but we have been sensitive to the issues of protecting this informality, whilst we simultaneously maintain a distant, but essential monitoring and evaluation of the meetings and so on.

Additionally, some members of the group have been asked to become more involved in various strands that are all vital to keeping it running, including becoming 'leaders'. Therefore, there is a process of evolution that maintains a healthy momentum at all times.

Our little group is not immune from the pressures of balancing the informal self-help world with the demands for democracy and accountability and 'transparency', but neither cancer and tragedy discriminate nor are they democratic, and so our structure is a blurred compromise; but it works.

It is my belief that to become obsessed with elements associated with democracy and accountability could easily lose potential volunteers and group members and a good process would be to surely start with enthusiastic people governed by a steering group and supervisory framework, such as that described in this chapter. As each separate group evolves, it would then develop its own individual structure that would be sensitive to the needs of its members and concurrently build its own framework.

However, obviously some governing structure is important so that you have some measurement available to make sure that relevant needs are being positively helped and addressed and that this help is easily accessible to all those who need it. Of course, most important of all, a coherent and recognizable referral system is essential, and someone has to manage that.

To summarize this section, we would suggest that the following features should be addressed, in one way or another, in establishing a new group:

- A structure of management, however loose, needs to be formulated. At the very least, this gives confidence to people like me and Angela who can contribute effectively in helping others as well as ourselves, and at all times feel supported. This is also very important for the practical purposes of providing the child-care because the volunteer organizers need to know at least approximately how many children they would be catering to.

- The existence of a hierarchy is very likely to be an attribute for a parent/carer group. It is a lonely and desolate time and most of those who have joined our group have very clearly stated that at least, initially, having semi-formal 'leaders' to guide them, relieved them of many more burdens at such a difficult time.

- A clear route for referrals needs to be prepared, with some kind of filtration system, so that people are not exposed too soon after a loss to what is potentially, if unintentionally an intrusive situation.

- A rolling record is helpful in knowing just who attended, and it is the practice in our group to take notes of each meeting, so that some continuity is preserved for big and little issues, since things easily get lost between meetings and in our own daily individual struggles.

- The core paradigm of the group is 'self-help', not user control and in any group that is established, we believe, it is important not to lose sight of what we are about to do.

Examples of individual anonymized 'grief histories'

Ralph

Ralph is a 46-year-old African-Caribbean man whose family originate in St Kitts. He has three children, two boys and a girl, and his wife died of leukaemia. He works in the fast food industry in a local chain of restaurants and has struggled to keep his job, his house, and his car. He has not received much help from the extended family either, on the maternal or paternal side, and he heard about the group through St Christopher's Hospice. On joining, he explained the struggles he had been having with almost every aspect of his life; but most of all he described the loneliness of his daily existence and the isolation that had engulfed him. He said that the others in the group had helped ease the terrible burdens of this loneliness and isolation, and made him feel less 'alone', especially in the sense that he was now in direct contact with those who could understand his predicament, even without him having to say anything.

After becoming a regular attender, Ralph told all of us how he had found even 'being there' and being soothed just by empathy was often enough to 're-charge his batteries'—so sometimes, he would merely sit quietly and listen to the struggles of some of the others who were struggling with their own loss. At other times, he would actively contribute, but he had said that for him the group had been a vital component in the complex machinery that had allowed most of us to recover from tragedy.

Perhaps most importantly, Ralph acknowledged that whilst we had been a remarkably resilient species, in some ways, he had found it very difficult, as a bereaved man, to seek out help, and he himself had been amazed as to how quickly he felt safe and comfortable even on his first attendance.

Rebecca

Rebecca, a white woman in her thirties, was never married to her partner, but they had been living together for a very long time and had a 12-year-old son. She works in a local library. Her partner committed suicide when there no indications that anything at all had been wrong. She described the utter desolation she had felt after the tragedy, of being overwhelmed by her own guilt in that she had not detected any signs that might have alerted her to her partner's hidden turmoil, and given her an opportunity to prevent him taking his own life.

Attempting to manage her own turbulent cocktail of thoughts had been difficult enough, but she described in the group, the almost impossibly sad task of trying to deal with her son's feelings, when she herself was barely able to function well. Rebecca said of the group that it was, 'the only place I have been able to come that deals with the parents on a self-help basis...that is what I need and what I am just not used to dealing with things on my own and that is why I come to the group as well, as others have said, you feel so much less alone'.

Regarding helping to understand the needs of her son, and to tolerate his challenges after her partner's death, she said the group had helped her keep her difficulties with her son in perspective, realizing that the repercussions of losing a partner had certain universal features in young children, whatever may be the cause of the death. She added that the gaps between the meetings, for her, allowed a 'yardstick' to measure her own recovery and adjustment, and to discuss with others how each person found his own pathway to this same process.

Gregory

Gregory is a white man in his forties; working in the oil technology field, with three children, two girls and one boy. His wife died after a very long illness, and for the last years of her life, she had been very disabled; including being wheelchair-bound. Gregory attended the group remarking that it had been the only arena where he had felt safe in expressing the jumble of emotions that erupted unexpectedly after his wife had died.

He candidly described an overwhelming sense of relief at her death, and the guilt that came with the feeling, a sense of relief, at the end of the suffering for his wife and for him and for his children. He said that these thoughts had deeply troubled him and at times he had been disgusted with himself, but after being able to express them in the group had given him a significant sense of release and relief.

Effectively, Gregory had been raising the children for a number of years with the help of the extended family, and also with professional child-care support. However, his demanding job and caring for his wife and children, and being supported by the extended family had, he noted, 'suppressed and suffocated my own life and sometimes I wished it was all over for my wife so we could all just get on with our lives...I felt appalled that I could think those things and here is the only place I have felt safe to let all of this out'.

Being a member of the group had helped him realign the 'jumble of emotions' described earlier and had enabled him to begin to rebuild his family life, at least partially freed from the haunting bonds of guilt that had been tormenting and repressing him for a significant period of time, both during his wife's illness, and after her death.

Amaryllis

Amaryllis is an African-Caribbean woman in her late thirties and she was born in Dominica, but came to the UK when she was seven years old. She comes from a strongly religious Catholic family whilst her parents have remained in her birth country, and her elderly maternal grandparents who raised her are in the UK. Her grandparents are in poor health. It was always the intention of her own parents and her two sisters to join the family in this country, but commercial success in Dominica in the cut-flower industry prevented this from happening. The family have remained close, and make frequent business, and holiday trips to the UK.

She has two children, an older teenage boy and a younger daughter, and her husband died of a rare form of blood cancer. She is employed as a financial controller in a small local factory making electrical components.

Amaryllis' husband had suffered a long illness, and the children had received a large amount of support from the local hospice, because they were finding it very difficult to see their father succumbing to the effects of the cancer; and also because they were worried about their mother. On top of all of this, the children were concerned about their grandparents in this country. When her husband died, both the children became sullen and withdrawn, and the situation was made unintentionally even more tense with the arrival of the extended family from Dominica, who tried to help, but their religious perspective just made things worse. Amaryllis felt that her own grief was being ignored in this scenario, and she found the group offered a space for herself, among people immersed in not dissimilar tragedies, and also with some members who were also struggling with extended families.

She felt she could safely 'dump' all her feelings 'on the table' in the meetings, and she said she also felt it was a safe place to candidly talk about her past relationship, which was at times, stormy and unhappy. She also said that the group was a place where she could openly say that—at times the deluge of help received by the children made her angry and jealous at times of stress. She also felt that the hypocrisy shown by some family members about the quality of her relationship and marriage after her husband's death was hurtful, almost as if they had wanted her to die because he was the better person. With so many emotions flying around, Amaryllis said the group was also a place where all these things could be discussed in an informal, friendly atmosphere, among people who not only understood the tensions of bereavement, but were themselves experiencing, or had experienced like situations.

Sandra

Sandra has three children and her husband had died suddenly of an illness that was never fully understood. She joined the group because she wanted to be among those who had been experiencing similar difficulties. She is a white middle class woman from a professional background who had unexpectedly found her two boys 'going off the rails' as she described it.

She said she had come from an high-achieving comfortable environment and devastating as her and her family's loss was, she thought she could deal with it all. She openly told the group how wrong she had been and how her two adolescent boys had become difficult and challenging, after their father's death. She said, in one group meeting, 'never in my wildest dreams did I think I would be fishing any of my children out of a police station at 2 am in the morning because they had been caught vandalizing property at a railway station'.

To be able to talk about this in our group had been an immense help to her, and had caused her to reconsider her own vulnerabilities and needs in relation to herself, as well as her family. She said the group absolved her of feelings of 'guilt' regarding having failed her children, and made her realize she was not a 'superwoman' and that her children needed help and so did she. She said that for her, the group was a catalyst for change and was a very positive experience.

Boundary setting, assimilation, and direction

How does the group recruit and assimilate new members who may be at different points of adjustment post-bereavement?

As a white, relatively elderly father with two young boys at the time we formed the group, paired with a young African-Caribbean mother with a young boy and girl, we hoped that this would be a good start-up combination as facilitators, to capture the broadest cross-section of people who might come to the group.

The group provides a quiet and safe time, away from children, where issues and feelings can be discussed openly in a confidential and supportive atmosphere among people who are united by personal trauma and tragedy.

The main aim of the group is to try and offer a forum and space for developing a self-support framework, where everything can be discussed without feeling stupid or silly.

Sensitivity to the different stages that people are in, is vital and we keep learning as we grow to tackle the variety of different things that people attending bring to the meetings, and we also keep learning the processes needed for the group when new people join, and others leave, and also when some drop in and drop out and drop in again.

The hospice is the main coordinating mechanism in assessing and referring people to the group, and I and Angela are given a brief description of each prospective joiner's circumstances, including how they lost their partner and the ages of the children, and so on. Additionally, if there are special areas of sensitivity or concern, we will be alerted.

This 'funnelling' process of assessing and referral is therefore undertaken within the professional arena and at the moment, we do not take self referrals. One reason for not accepting self-referrals is that the professional 'funnel' preserves a source of qualified expertise, if situations arise, that may need expert intervention.

Each session begins with introductions, even if we all know one another, we can forget in the gaps between meetings, and if new people have joined we give them time to talk about their circumstances, and how long it had been since their partner had died. However, some have not wanted to do this until they felt comfortable in doing so, and it is important to recognize obviously that we all have different vulnerabilities.

A particularly raw area is when relatively newly bereaved people join the group, and listen to others talk about wanting or having new relationships, or perhaps confessing that actually they had an awful relationship with their deceased partner—this scenario can be distressing and tense, if it is insensitively managed and can result in an exclusion rather than an assimilation-process occurring.

In our group, we try and regularly mention this feature of bereavement, so that we do not unintentionally upset others when the 'rawness' of loss and death has become diluted, as time separates us from our own tragedies.

The dynamics of this type of self-help group are daunting and complex, but we try to be as aware and sensitive as we can, so as to be able to cater to as many people as possible who might want something a bit different from one another at any one time.

Inevitably, a 'core' group has been formed from those who nearly always appear for meetings, but we have been as aware as we can, in not allowing an informal hierarchy to emerge within the group between the regulars and the not so regulars, and in particular, we have loose rules to make as certain as possible that newcomers feel welcome and assimilated into the entire process; as it would be all too easy to feel excluded, if you are new and vulnerable and hear others talk seemingly casually about heart-break and tragedy.

Most of the assimilation process is social common sense, built around a loose structure as suggested above. The following points may be of guidance to others:

◆ Our experience would suggest that it is very important to have a professional referral and assessment process to ensure that people are ready and prepared to be exposed to a group.

◆ A professional system also allows a process of evaluation and monitoring to occur. We do not want accidentally to do more harm than good. Neither is it safe to assume that because it is self-help, it is automatically good. We want to achieve a positive outcome for those attending but there must be some accountability within the informal framework, as 'self-help' should not dissolve into 'self-righteous'. This could be a significant risk, if there is no professional linkage.

◆ It is important to have a process of introduction at each session to help all those involved to know where they are on the bereavement spectrum. As noted in this chapter, it is essential **not** to unintentionally shock or upset newcomers.

◆ Be aware of cultural and religious and class issues.

◆ Be aware of gender issues in setting up a group and while attracting referrals and assimilating new people. The gender imbalance in the professional bereavement services is startling and it is important not to replicate this process in a self-help setting. It would appear to be important to mix class, gender, and ethnicity to attract a similarly balanced clientele.

◆ A mechanism for following up new referrals who do not continue is very helpful in developing a group, and monitoring the assimilation process. This is another advantage of having access to professional expertise.

How participants' common needs and different needs determine the length of individual attendance at the group

Within our own histories of grief, we all have unique experiences of tragedy and reconstruction and the self-help group has effectively allowed us all a forum to express our individual grief paradigm and to seek equally individual succour from our involvement.

For many of us struggling to raise our children on our own, being part of the group has become a continuum, where we compare notes and disasters about our children, our in-laws, about Christmas, and about holidays, and about love and loss.

For some, there is a specific motive; an example is a young woman, who attended just once. She had been widowed about eighteen months previously and had developed a relationship with a new man and was immersed in and confused by the chemistry of the feelings and emotions that buffeted her, at this time in her life. She attended the group and explained her feelings and clearly sought redemption and release from the turmoil that was holding her back—she said listening to others helped her sort out her dilemmas.

Some attenders have found new relationships but remained in the group, while others have not. And the others, with older children have left when these children have passed into adulthood.

A number of people drop in and out of the group. One man said he felt that it was really helpful to him to know that the group was there and he could just turn up, if he felt like it, at a particular time.

He said he had found no other source of support that could offer this, and that did not make him feel guilty, if he just did not feel like turning up at a particular session. He added that it was also comfortable to be in a group where there are other men.

To encompass as many people as possible, it is difficult to provide guidelines as to the length of stay, and the process of evolution should in itself determine the direction each individual self-help group takes. In our own group, we are developing as we go, but if the numbers who attend go above eighteen, we have arranged to divide them into two groups, for two thirds of each session, coming together for the last third.

Two informal facilitators/users would join the separated units. If the number of referrals grows significantly, and those regularly attending also continues to grow, we have developed plans to start to build up a second group.

Rules including potential child protection issues and mental health issues

Although informal, the following guidelines have been agreed upon for the group and the main points are available in a leaflet that is sent to those referred. They include the following:

♦ All those involved are told that if there are significant child protection or mental health concerns, we will bring this to the attention of our hospice's social work service. This is a further reason for an attachment to a formal professional structure;

♦ No discrimination of any form;

♦ Respect for others and allow everyone to have their own time to talk;

♦ To try and be on time;

- All information except the issue in the first bullet point is confidential;
- Friends cannot attend in support.

Topic Agenda

Examples of topics that regularly emerge in sessions:

- Practical issues such as state benefits, and the lack of them
- The political agenda around single parenthood or lone parenthood
- The awfulness of state education and health service
- Children growing up, their sexuality and how we deal with it as lone parents
- Adjusting to grief and loss and the individual processes we all develop to adapt ourselves to our post-bereavement world
- Having feelings about possible new relationships and how we deal with the guilt that it sometimes arises. How do we tell our children if we want to start a new relationship?
- How do we know if our children are being naughty or just normal? Are they reacting to grief and loss, or are they just being normal, horrible little beasts?
- Sometimes we talk about the seemingly relentless sadness and loneliness that we all experience at one time or the other. This is often a powerful force in the group's cohesion—we explore these feelings and sometimes lighten them with humour and optimism that can be grim and determined, or light-hearted and flippant—but the commonalty of these intensely focused emotions is, we believe, where the group derives much of its strength, which flows back to the members and hopefully boosts the individual survival techniques most of us develop after tragedy.

Summary

Our group has now been running since November 1999 and usually ten to sixteen people attend each session, and we meet about six times per year. We have formal child-care supported sessions which number three, each year. The logistics of organizing these supported sessions is formidable, involving volunteer drivers, volunteer child care workers, and also paid support from a section of the hospice including administrative help with post, and so on. However formidable as it sounds and as it is, it has been accomplished, but as noted earlier in this chapter, it is vital to have some form of organizational and administrative infrastructure so that precious and dedicated volunteer time is not wasted, for instance, it is unhelpful to expect twenty children and only have six turn up because there is no system in place to estimate who is actually likely to turn up.

Apart from the formal supported sessions, we now have four other gatherings during the year; we usually have two picnics or a visit to a theme park and a Christmas party.

Generally, we have maintained a very diverse ethnic class and gender mix, and indeed the number of men attending regularly is now equal to the women and as a man I have found this aspect particularly beneficial. Single parenthood is usually associated with women, and to a certain extent choice, and can be contaminated with guilt for being part of a non-nuclear family—all of these things can be safely discussed and/or disposed within our group.

We have people who are unemployed, we have people who are employed in catering, in the health and social care professions, in industry, in office work, and in teaching and we have a musician and a financial adviser and a gas fitter engineer amongst our group. This diversity seems to lead to an equality of contributions from all those who attend.

Usually we take notes or minutes at each formal session to keep a loose continuity, but they also serve as a semi-formal method for us to begin evaluation as to how we ourselves are functioning and to see if things that regularly arise are just not being addressed or dealt with.

Perhaps most importantly, we believe we have been able to establish a network based on self-help but framed by professional hospice staff, to rescue those parents and carers like Angela and I, who are at the risk of being overwhelmed by the chaos and sadness and mixed emotions that rage around us at such a vulnerable and lonely time.

Because bad luck and tragedy do not discriminate, amongst those who attend, we are bound to have one or two people who present challenges through personality problems or other difficulties that may have little association with their bereavement, or perhaps their bereavement exacerbates these underlying fault-lines. Usually the group process can contain such situations, and so far any such manifestations in our group have only been lightweight, but clearly any group should have a strategy for containing and cushioning possible 'problem' people who may not respect conventional boundaries.

The security of the professional framework serves many purposes including providing support in situations as noted above; but particularly for the facilitators, it provides a measure of boundary setting and a vital access link for psychological and social work support for those that the group believes are in need of extra, more formal assistance, or containment. We hope the group provides sustenance to the bereaved parents and carers at a desolate and lonely time, and afterwards as well. Perhaps, it makes us more reflective and better parents, which in turn makes our children more thoughtful and adaptive to our individual tragedies. Perhaps, it helps us not just to salvage what we can from the wreckage but to reconstruct positively. But we are sure of one thing, that at the very least, the group provides one route to safely share our own histories of grief.

Endpiece

As I come to the end of writing this chapter on my Caribbean holiday, I watch the sun slip toward the horizon, glowing like a huge red Rowntree's fruit pastille. The old wooden boat and the impossible number of pelicans squeezed on its deck are bathed by the Rowntree's light. Suddenly the birds take flight–a camera man appears out of the red, followed by people carrying flowers which they shower on a couple on the beach. It is their twenty-fifth wedding anniversary and their friends have organized this surprise flower attack!

It is almost exactly twenty years since I came to this tropic with Susan, and I look at the happy anniversary couple glowing red in the sunset, deliriously and deliciously confused victims of the flower-assault. They hug each other and their friends, and of course I think what might have been for us. But I am not blue in the red sunset; although my world will now always have a shade of sadness, since losing Susan, the

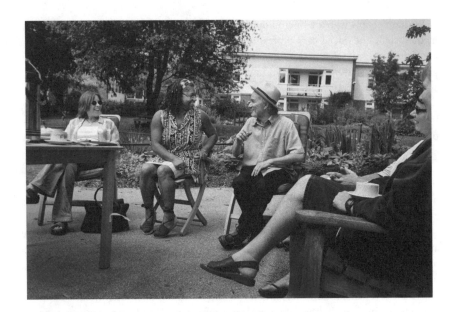

enormous difference is that I think what can still be, and I would not be in that place, if it were not for all the formal and informal help my family has received.

Dedicated to the memory of Susan Dennison and Sean Paul, and the history of the future

I have been greatly assisted in the writing of this chapter by Angela Paul. Her regal ability to balance a healthy indiffernce to formality and bureaucracy, with her infectious qualities of calm, conhesiveness, and practicality has been an enduringly beneficial component of the group.

Index